All About the Dobermann

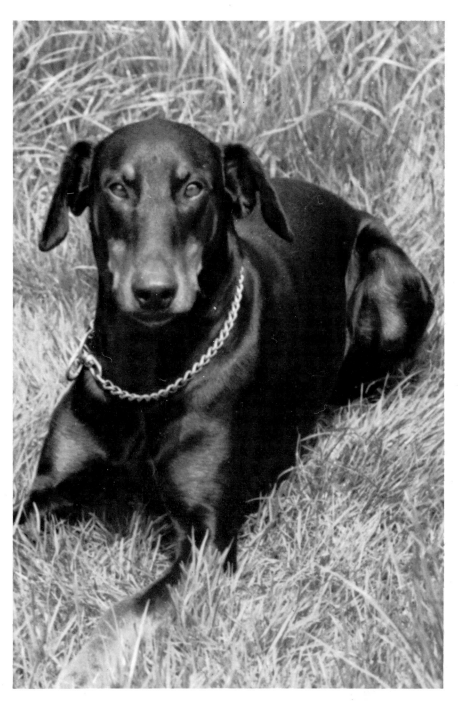

Frontispiece   Kelly – a once in a lifetime dog. How empty my life would have been if I had never known him.

All about the Dobermann

jan Irven

PELHAM BOOKS

First published in Great Britain by
Pelham Books Ltd
27 Wrights Lane
London W8 5TZ
1986
Reprinted 1986

© 1986 by jan Irven

Irven, jan
    All about the Dobermann.
    1. Dobermann pinschers
    I. Title
    636.7'3   SF429.P5

    ISBN 0-7207-1639-X

Typeset, printed and bound by
Butler & Tanner Ltd, Frome and London

Contents

Acknowledgements

The author would like to thank the following people for their help in compiling this book: Mr Wyssmann, President of the Swiss Dobermann Club; F. Striby, President and Madeleine Gueit, Secretary of the Dobermann Club of France; Avi Marshak, Israel Chairman of the Israel Dobermann Club; Madeline George, President of the Puerto Rican Dobermann Club; George Jan Kranen, Secretary of The Dobermann Club Netherlands; Dr A. Hudono, Indonesia; Nancy Christensen, USA; Takashi Wakao, Japan; Joanna Walker & Joy, USA; Pat Bolton and Biddy Rowland for their help on the psychology of the Dobermann; Alma and Martin Page – Findjans Kennels for their tremendous help and advice; The Kennel Club for permission to reproduce the Breed Standard; Rex Hodge; Robert Elliott my vet, for his time, effort and immense help and work on the entire veterinary section of this book; Peter Austin – special thanks for the cover picture and private photographs in this book.

The extract from *Training Dogs* by Konrad Most is reproduced by permission of the author and Hutchinson Publishing Group Ltd.

Very special thanks to Ann Stone who gave unstintingly of her time and the contribution of the line drawings and sincere and grateful thanks to everyone else who responded to my requests and contributed so willingly with the many photographs.

To all my friends who gave me the confidence and inspiration to write this book I say a very big 'thank you' and last but not least to my very special husband George, without whose patience, encouragement and faith in me, I could never have succeeded.

The author and the publishers are grateful to the following to reproduce copyright photographs in this book:

John L. Ashbey page 84; Margaret Bastable 2; Roger Chambers 76; Ruth Clements 75; Frank Garwood 22; H. Grunig 85; Dr A. Hudono 88; The Kennel Club (figs 1, 2 and 3) 26 and 27; Larry and Cheri McNealy 91; Diane Pearce 17 (bottom), 71; James Tolleth 17 (top), 45; Heidi Vyse 64; Mrs S. Wilson 9. In some cases it has not been possible to ascertain the copyright holder and it is hoped that any such omissions will be excused.

Author's Preface

I decided to write this book very early on in my time as Secretary to the Dobermann Club. Apart from the fact that I was being inundated with questions, problems and requests for general information about the breed there was no one book that I could really recommend, that would not tie someone down with lots of technical and complicated reading. It was clear to me then that the problems I was being presented with by the general public, who were eager to buy a Dobermann, were those which should never have occurred. When I realised what was happening to my beloved breed, through sheer ignorance and lack of information, the idea for this book was born.

A Dobermann is a very special dog, a breed of dog that does not like to be mishandled. He is not a dog for everyone and in the wrong hands and with unsuitable environment and upbringing this breed of dog can be very dangerous.

There has been an alarming increase in the number of Dobermanns bred and those registered at the Kennel Club – 1978: 2097; 1979: 3107; 1980: 4634; 1981: 4824, 1982: 6244; 1983: 8499; 1984: 8905 – are only the tip of the iceberg. The number bred and not registered is a frightening thought. If left unchecked then unscrupulous, uncaring or uninformed breeders out to supply demand can do a great deal of harm and set back progress knowledgeable breeders have attained in stabilising and enhancing the breed. Eliminating the market for mass produced Dobermanns will go a long way in maintaining quality.

Because of the size and temperament of the Dobermann, it is obvious that temperament should be of paramount importance and the knowledge of what is behind each pedigree only comes from years of experience.

Apart from the inexperienced people breeding the Dobermann these same people are selling the puppies to the wrong types of owners. Because so many puppies are being sold that are weak and sickly – from some dubious puppy farmer, pet shop or irresponsible breeder – they start their little lives badly because they are never out of the vets and are often abandoned because the owner just cannot afford the vet fees. There are hundreds of reasons for not wanting to keep a Dobermann puppy and it is always the dog which suffers. They are pushed from pillar to post and in many cases badly treated and all because the breeder did not care enough to find the right type of home and to see that the people were responsible, caring and suitable to own a Dobermann.

For many of the new owners, the joy of owning their first Dobermann puppy has been marred, often by tragedy. They find out that although they have bought in good faith, they have bought a sick puppy and as has been the case in several instances the puppy has been so ill it has had to be put to sleep, a traumatic experience for someone who perhaps has saved up all their pennies to buy the puppy.

Badly bred puppies are often destined to grow up in the wrong environment because the commercial breeders have not cared about finding the right home. This then becomes a vicious circle.

I am painting a very black picture of what is happening but until both the breeders and the prospective owners of Dobermanns are more careful about buying and selling puppies this problem will never be resolved.

I know first hand how many people are frightened because the puppy grows bigger than they imagined and growls when it plays. They think they have a vicious puppy on their hands and because they play rough and are too playful, the new owner cannot cope and then they panic and decide they cannot keep the puppy. Or the puppy is left alone for hours on end and becomes restless, bored, naughty, unhappy and starts to destroy whatever it can. In some instances the puppy has not been cared for properly and not house-trained. Young puppies of six months old have been put to sleep because the owner did not have the time, patience or inclination to train the puppy to be house clean.

New owners or would be owners should really study the breed in depth and talk to lots of people who own Dobermanns before embarking on buying a Dobermann puppy.

Because of my desperate love for the breed and its well being this book is my contribution to try and bring the explosion of the Dobermann population under control. Leave the breeding to the experienced and hope the popularity of the Dobermann will die down and revert back to being a breed of which to be proud.

Of course there are many people who buy a Dobermann for the first time and are hooked on the breed and do everything that is right with the knowledge that is available to them, but for every person who buys one puppy there are six who buy from the wrong sources and are the wrong type of owners.

I have tried to write clearly for the first time owner of the Dobermann and to put down in an easily understood book, the joys, delights and happiness that comes from owning a Dobermann.

I have also tried to point out the pitfalls that can and do happen and for anyone thinking of buying a Dobermann for the first time I hope that they will read this book and learn from it and the mistakes made by others.

Learn to understand the breed first, there are so many other aspects of the Dobermann besides breeding, help to promote the breed by wise and careful consideration of the Dobermann, they are most definitely a breed to nurture and cherish. And finally learn to understand the way they behave and what makes them tick – this is what owning a Dobermann is all about.

POWER OF THE DOG

There is sorrow enough in the natural way,
From men and women to fill our day,
Yet when we are certain of sorrow in store,
Why do we always arrange for more?
Brothers and sisters I bid you beware,
of giving your hearts to a dog to tear.

Buy a pup and your money will buy,
Love unflinching that cannot lie,
Perfect passion and worship fed
By a kick in the ribs or a pat on the head.
Nevertheless it is hardly fair,
To risk your heart for a dog to tear.

When the fourteen years which nature permits
are closing in asthma or tumour or fits,
And the vet's unspoken prescriptions runs
to lethal chambers, or loaded guns,
Then you will find it's your own affair
But you've given your heart to a dog to tear.

When that body that lived at your single will,
When the whimper of welcome is stilled (how still!!)
When the spirit that answered your every mood
Is gone – wherever it goes – for good,
You still discover how much you care,
And will give your heart to a dog to tear.

We've sorrow enough in the natural way
When it comes to burying Christian clay
Our loves are not given but only lent,
At compound interest of cent per cent,
Though it is always the case, I believe
That the longer we've kept them the more we grieve,
For when debts are payable, right or wrong,
A short time loan is as bad as a long –
So why in heaven (before we go there)
Should we give our hearts to a dog to tear?

Rudyard Kipling.

1 History of the Breed

Origin and development

The history of the Dobermann is intriguing and fascinating although rather steeped in mystery. No definite records were kept by the man who brought about this lovely breed. It is an intelligent assumption that several breeds were used in the evolution of the Dobermann.

Louis Dobermann of Apolda in Germany was a tax and rent collector during the 1880s, and he also had the advantage of being the keeper of the dog pound where all stray dogs within his area were sent. He was obviously an avid dog lover who had a penchant towards aggressive animals.

Many thoroughbred, crossbred and mongrel dogs came into Herr Dobermann's dog pound and he had in his mind a dog of average build, smooth short coat, and above all he wanted stamina, intelligence and alertness in his companion who would be travelling with him wherever he went on his tax collecting works.

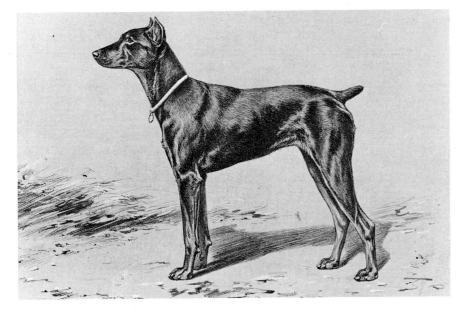

Norma Von Griessen 1909.

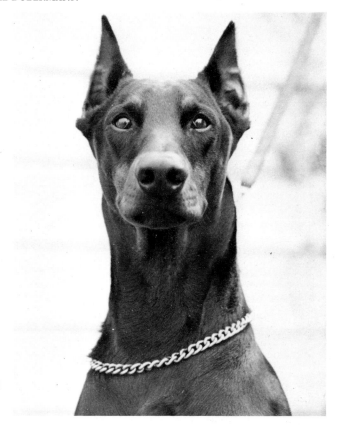

Wilm Von Forell.
Imported and owned
by Mrs M. Bastable
– Barrimilne.

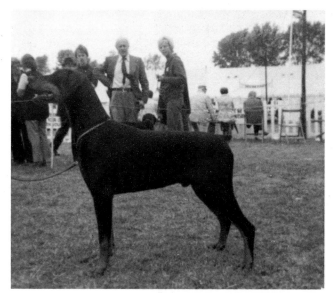

Ch Flexor
Flugleman won the
Working Group at
Crufts in 1975,
Winner of 15 C.C.s.
Bred and owned by
David Crick.

The German Pinscher was, according to photographs, a rather non-descript dog but he did have the reputation of being aggressive and alert and it was around this breed that Herr Dobermann built his dog.

The Germans had developed the ear cropping habit for certain breeds even in those far off days which was done to reduce the huge pendulous ears and make it difficult for other dogs to maintain a hold when fighting. From the date of the breed's inception up until the 1920's ears were cropped to a small size; more recently a larger crop has been adopted to add elegance to the head.

The Rottweiler did much to bring the Dobermann Pinscher into being and it was a credit to Herr Dobermann for his forethought of using such an intelligent dog in his bloodlines. It is also generally accepted that the Manchester Terrier was used in the evolution of the Dobermann and this is evident in the short, gleaming coat and distinctive black and tan markings, the use of the Manchester Terrier blood also did something towards the refinement and elegance.

Some French enthusiasts consider that Beauceron blood was used and this is very feasible because the Beauceron is a solid, upstanding dog, bright and alert. The Beauceron often carries a white patch on the chest which was apparent in the original Dobermanns and still crops up occasionally today. The Pointer could also have been used as if you watch a Dobermann exercising it will stop and point with the correct foreleg and tailset. The Greyhound was almost certainly used because of its height, stamina and speed.

There is no shadow of a doubt that from 1900 to the present day the improvement in type has been tremendously progressive, with excellent dogs in almost every country but there are also many that do not fit the correct standard of the breed.

Herr Goeller who also came from Apolda was the man who took up the breed where Herr Dobermann left off. An improvement in quality was noticed in the late 19th Century but it was in Apolda where the breed originated that the evolution really took place.

From the beginning black and brown Dobermanns were being born but it was not until 1906 that the first blue dog appeared. It would appear that there was no objection to this new colour so it was included in the standard. Careful breeding programmes adopted by responsible breeders in Germany helped to standardise type and overall refinement of the Dobermann.

At this time several kennels in Switzerland and Holland had been established and were working to a careful breeding programme. It was in 1912 that the first Isabella coloured Dobermann was born in Germany. Sadly the breeding stock in Germany was depleted by 1918 and until 1922 no real recovery was made. A gradual improvement in quality was made in the next three to four years when Americans came to Germany and in 1926 acquired many of the best dogs. In 1899 Otto Goeller organised a National Dobermann Pinscher Club and one year later he and other enthusiasts drew up the Standard. Official recognition by the German Kennel Club was immediately obtained. Apart from height and one or two minor alterations relating to conformation there has been little change in the Standard adopted in all countries.

Dobermanns in Britain

Little was known about the breed before 1948 and there were less than half a dozen registered over here before the 1939 war. Several importations were made in 1947, mainly from Europe; the Dobermann Club was formed in 1948 and by 1951 some two hundred Dobermanns had been registered.

The police began to take notice of this new breed which was being used successfully by forces abroad and Dobermanns entered the police force, notably in Surrey and Durham, in 1949. Although Dobermanns were used successfully the police still favour the German Shepherd Dog.

In the early days, the Birling and Tavey prefixes led the field but other historic names followed – Cartergate, Sonhende, Triogen, Trevillis, Barrimilne and Tumlow to name a few – all of which played a great part in producing the lines of today.

With the explosion in recent times of the Dobermann population it would be impossible to quote all the kennel names that successfully appear in the show ring, in fact under current revised Kennel Club regulations, prefixes and suffixes are no longer readily available and must be won in the show ring at Championship Level by winning, first, second or third place in post graduate class with a dog bred by yourself.

To anyone interested in the breed's well being, the present increase in numbers can only be alarming when registrations are now eight thousand plus per annum, and many others in addition are not registered. Since 1980 there has been an alarming increase in the number of Dobermanns bred and it has reached absolute saturation point. The price for the puppies has hit an all time high and demand still outstrips the supply. Commercial people jumping on the bandwagon, realising the prices the breed demands, are acquiring bitches one way or the other and breeding as often as they can but never worrying whether the puppies will find good permanent homes, and many sell whole litters to dealers up and down the country. This mass breeding alarms the breeders who breed solely to improve the breed and the Rescue Service is sadly overworked with dogs and bitches coming on to Rescue as early as eight to nine weeks, and many of only just six months have been rehoused several times.

In spite of what some devotees feel and say, the Dobermann was produced to be, and still should be, a working dog, although clearly it is not possible for all owners to have the wish or the facilities to work them. All Dobermanns should be bred to have the working capability – adherence to the Breed Standard would largely ensure this. Too many 'breeders' appear either to ignore the Standard or to see how it can be interpreted to justify their own whims. Hence the wide variety of types seen at present.

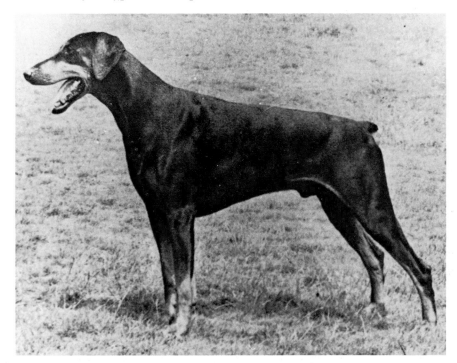

Ch Tumlow Satan. Bred by Mr & Mrs R. Harris. Owned by George Collins. Twice Best of Breed at Crufts.

Temperament and character are all important – as a famous Austrian breeder who was also that country's foremost veterinary professor adamantly said 'with a faulty construction you will not get the correct temperament'. There is no reason why strength and elegant beauty cannot be combined, would anyone deny, that in his prime Mohammed Ali possessed both to a remarkable degree?

The full Breed Standard will be found on page 136 in Appendix 2.

2   Character of the Dobermann

'The Dobermann is a dog of good medium size, with a well set body, muscular and elegant. He has a proud carriage and a bold and alert temperament. His form is compact and tough and owing to his build, capable of great speed. His gait is light and elastic, his eyes show intelligence and firmness of character and he is loyal and obedient. Shyness or viciousness must be heavily penalised.' This is what is said about the Dobermann in the Breed Standard and this is what it must be.

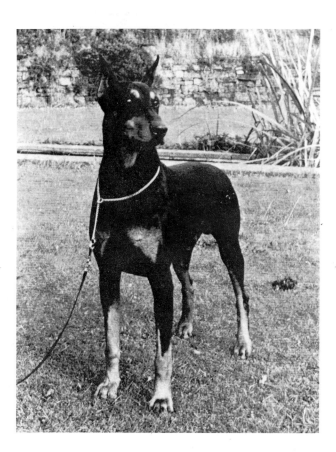

Vanessa's Little Dictator of Tavey. Bred by Mr E. Edgar & Mrs B. Garner. Owned by Mrs J. Curnow.

Temperament

Some dogs are known for their gentleness, while others, through no fault of their own, develop very bad reputations and the Dobermann is a breed that unfortunately has such a reputation. They are a type of dog which needs to be treated with great respect. They are smart dogs and do not like to be mishandled. Dobermanns love their masters and immediate family and want to protect everything dear to them.

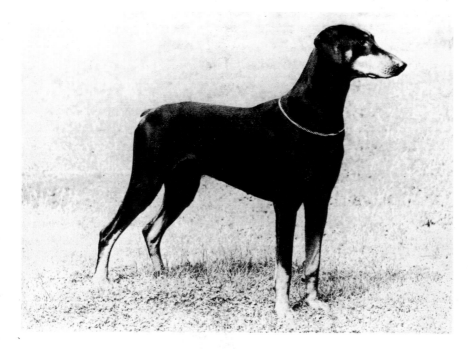

Ch Iceberg of Tavey. Bred by Mrs J. Curnow & Miss E. Would. Owned by Mrs J. Curnow. Winner of 33 C.C.s.

A Dobermann needs love and affection as much as any animal but the Dobermann rewards affection with devotion which is second to none. The closeness that a master feels for his dog and the dog for his master is a bond which is unbreakable. People who own a Dobermann are never really satisfied with any other breed, the fanatical loyalty inherent in this breed is visible from the very first time you bring your puppy home and Dobermanns just love to be with you in everything you do. Your Dobermann will be your constant companion, even when you are in a foul mood he will still feel the same about you.

Alertness is his most dominant characteristic and he is aware all the time of what is going on around. He may be sleeping stretched out, his head on his paws dozing, but he knows exactly where you are. When I am out running my dogs, my dog runs ahead and you would think he was far too busy to even remember he was out with me. The bitches stay closer to me and all the time the three of them are running and sniffing they are turning their heads to see where I am.

The Dobermann welcomes you and the family home, even after only a short while left on his own, with joy and pleasure, his eyes sparkling with happiness, his mouth in a big happy Dobermann grin, his teeth showing big and white and his little tan bum and stumpy tail wagging and wobbling like jelly on a plate.

A Dobermann also has a great sense of humour, some actually do grin when they play their little jokes on you, my old Kelly always bites my bottom when he is happy and playful.

Dobermanns to me are to be likened to a beautiful dressage horse, so full of elegance, grace and dignity, the strength and balance of the breed makes the comparison obvious.

Unfortunately, Dobermanns do have a bad reputation. People who have not known a Dobermann always say 'Aren't they supposed to be fierce, unpredictable and vicious?' Unfortunately with more and more people breeding and jumping on the bandwagon this has got to happen, but if newcomers were more selective in their choice of breeder and avoided puppy farms, pet shops and dubious breeders and looked into the whole aspect of buying a dog more thoroughly, perhaps the mass breeding would slow down.

Temperament is paramount in this breed – it has got to be, nowadays the dogs are in a lot of cases bigger than the Standard calls for. When thoughtless and inexperienced people turn their hand to breeding, dubious puppies frequently result. Often they do not realise or care to acknowledge that strength and muscle combined with bad temperament in the stud dog – mated on to a bitch with an equally bad temperament – will most likely result in puppies with unreliable temperaments.

Mating Dobermann to Dobermann without consulting the pedigrees of both dog and bitch to see if they match well is just asking for trouble. Trouble that need never occur if dogs are properly bred, handled and sold to the right homes. To see tough men, women and teenagers strutting along with a Dobermann wearing an enormous spiked collar, on a short lead, the dog snorting and snarling and aggressive is not what the Dobermann is all about.

A Dobermann is not a bully and neither is he mean but if he should be attacked by another dog or even another human being then he will fight, usually with very sad results for the opponent.

To sum up, the Dobermann is a powerful, alert, intelligent and devoted companion, honest and trustworthy with unequalled loyalty.

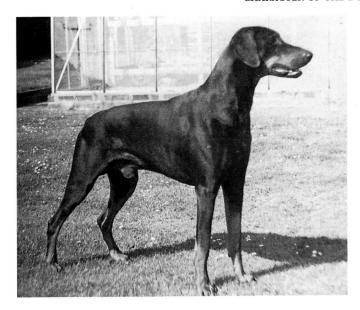

Ch Olderhill Sherboygan. Bred and owned by Mrs S. Wilson. Made breed history, together with his sister Olderhill Sioux, when they won both the dog C.C. and bitch C.C. twice. They are the only litter brother and sister owned, bred and handled by the same person to do so.

The Dobermann is a character all his own, never equalled in any other breed, he is breathtakingly beautiful and courageous and will guard you with his life, no matter how soppy he may appear in daily life, that instinct is there and will come to the surface when needed. So for all he has to offer us the very least we can do for him is to treat him with love and respect and make his life as happy as he makes ours.

Take care of your Dobermann, precious thing that he is, and if the time ever comes when you have to part with him, for whatever reason, don't give him away to anyone who could abuse him, get in touch with the breeder to help you or get in touch with Dobermann Rescue who are very experienced in finding happy homes for lonely, often ill-treated and unwanted Dobermanns.

As this book has been written for the newcomer to the breed and will hopefully act as a guide I thought perhaps a section on the current dogs who have made an impact on the breed would be useful. So many newcomers go along and look at puppies and haven't the faintest idea when shown a pedigree what it is all about. Throughout this book are some of the outstanding dogs in this country over the last decade. These dogs have been dominant stud dogs and brood bitches and the puppies being bred today will more often than not carry these lines.

Psychology of the Dobermann

Today the adult male Dobermann can be quite a handful and has been likened by some to a loaded gun. Being such a fast and powerfully built animal, it is important that the adult Dobermann does not become over-dominant. Dominance is a more common problem amongst males than bitches and it is so very important that Dobermanns are sensibly raised by reasonably competent owners. Thoughtless spoiling and 'giving in' to lovely little puppies all too often leads to unmanageable hooligan adults.

A sensibly raised Dobermann who is a much loved companion will often form a very close and almost telepathic bond with his owner. Most Dobermanns are trustworthy with friendly strangers, but it is not unusual for them to be rather aloof, uninterested or even actively dislike being approached by strangers, and their suspicions are easily aroused by what seems to them unusual or startling actions.

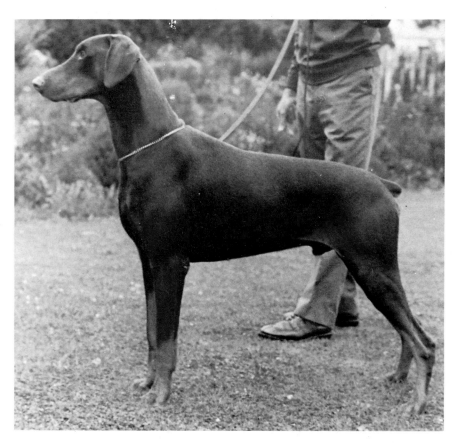

Phileens Duty Free of Tavey.

Some Dobermanns accused of being 'shy' are merely affronted by complete strangers rushing up and expecting to be greeted like long lost friends before they have even had time to do the usual sniff and inspection. The Dobermann likes to make his own mind up as to whether he wants to be friendly or not and does not like to be pushed into playing the fool with 'outsiders'.

When the Dobermann is taken into the family, a 'pecking order' must be established so that the Dobermann is very clear who is 'boss'. If no direction is given to the pup as a youngster he may, if he is a naturally dominant character, try to take over as 'boss' himself. This is a most unhappy situation both for the Dobermann and for his unfortunate owner. The Dobermann is at his best and happiest with a strong loving owner whom he can respect and rely on, and he loses all sense of direction and purpose if allowed to run wild. Consistence and clarity are the most important things to remember in training the youngster.

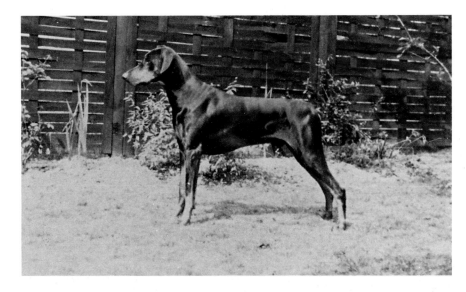

Ch Findjans Poseidon. Bred and owned by Mr & Mrs Page. Winner of 8 C.C.s, 13 R.C.C.s, J.W. Sire of 14 Champions, Top Stud Dog U.K.

The Dobermann is very eager to learn and to please his owner but can only do so if he understands what is required of him. With the young pup the owner takes the place of the bitch - watch a bitch and her pups, she is always alert and aware, giving them lots of physical love and attention, but punishing transgressions immediately and forcefully.

Praise should be given immediately every time the dog does something well or pleases you in any way, and transgressions should be

noticed and dealt with immediately every time too (unless they occurred through your own negligence or unclear directions). Verbal
punishment is adequate in most circumstances but physical punishment may occasionally be necessary as a back-up especially during
the male's adolescent stage when he is testing his dominance. Allow
a dog to 'get away' with something once and it will be harder the next
time to correct him. I am sure much of the unwarranted aggression
seen all too often in adults is due to the laxity of owners in not
correcting the problem early on in the dog's development. A dog
should be discouraged at an early age from displaying unwarranted
aggression towards other dogs or people and learn that unpleasant
consequences follow if he doesn't behave himself. Far too many owners seem to think it amusing when their dogs 'fly out' at all and
sundry and bark and growl at others. It only needs a broken chain or
slipped leash for most unpleasant consequences to follow. After all,
the Dobermann is supposed to be a working dog and what good is a
working dog that cannot be controlled?

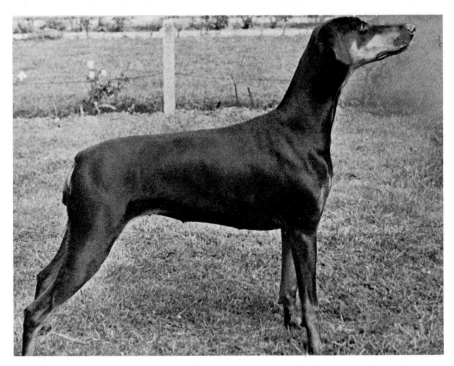

Ch Mitrasanda Gay
Lady of Findjans.
Bred by Mr & Mrs
Taylor. Owned by
Mr & Mrs Page.
Winner of 4 C.C.s,
2 R.C.C.s, J.W.
Dam of Ch
Poseidon.

Although there are general characteristics common to all Dobermanns, there is great variation amongst individuals. Generally speak-
ing the Dobermann is a late maturing dog and can (like humans) go

through a juvenile delinquent stage anytime between six or seven months up to about eighteen months old. This is more common with males. In bitches they sometimes go through a rather similar stage but become rather shy and unsure of themselves for a period, unlike the males who are more likely to be over-confident, bumptious and wilful.

By the time the Dobermann is getting over his adolescent stage he should be calming down and be fairly biddable and obedient. Most Dobermanns will live as family companions so it is most important that breeders aim towards breeding reasonably steady and reliable dogs which will be able to fulfil the role expected of them. Temperament leaves a lot to be desired in some Dobermanns and with the number of inexperienced owners coming into the breed this is not going to help the 'Rescue' situation. Most behavioural problems do stem from puppyhood when they are at their most impressionable, but breeders can do a lot to help by trying to keep in touch with novice owners and helping them through the early stages of ownership and training.

The puppy looks to his owner for guidance and confidence and a calm confident person will help to produce a calm and confident Dobermann. Never flap or fuss. If the pup growls or snaps at you, growl back and give him a quick spank or shake. Love him and talk to him and let him be with you as much as possible and you will build up a lasting and rewarding relationship. It is a tremendous responsibility to take on a Dobermann – you will be the centre of his world for as long as he lives and you must live up to the obligation that involves. Do not boss or bully – command him with firmness, confidence and consistency and he will give back all you expect. Most Dobermanns hate loud and high pitched noises, shouting and shrieking gets on their nerves as much as it gets on ours. They either get over excited and start barking and snapping or go into a sulk and retire to hide somewhere quiet until things quieten down.

One does come across the occasional over sensitive and nervous Dobermann. This is more common amongst bitches but can occur with either sex. The first signs usually appear at about seven weeks of age when the pup will start to run away and hide from visitors rather than come out and see them. This is the stage when pups start to differentiate between known 'family' and 'strangers'. Sometimes it is a fleeting stage, disappearing rapidly as the puppy becomes settled into a new home and starts to become more socialised. On the other hand it can hang on right through adolescence – but usually eventually improves with maturity and sensible socialisation and training. Shyness with people can be helped by taking the Dobermann into situations where there are lots of neutral people about and not letting people come rushing up to try and handle the dog. Most of these types will improve if they can be taken into situations where people will ignore them and then they eventually start to become inquisitive about people and will begin making tentative approaches on their own behalf. The main thing is to realise they do not like to be rushed but will come round if allowed to go at their own pace. Punishment is usually self defeating, as is over encouragement and over enthusiasm. The best thing is to train the Dobermann to sit quietly at your side when you stop and talk as they cannot wriggle and squirm out of the way if they have their bottom firmly on the ground.

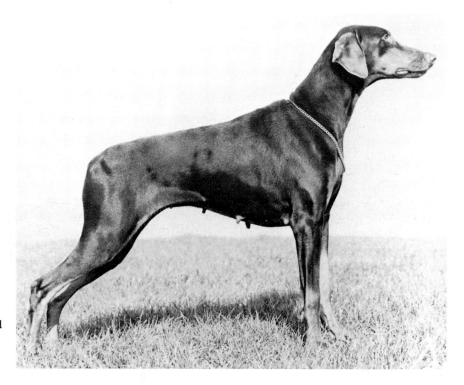

Ch Findjans Freya. Bred and owned by Mr & Mrs Page. Winner of 4 C.C.s, 3 R.C.C.s. Finished her show career by winning the Bitch C.C. at Crufts.

If you want to show a Dobermann that is nervous then do try only to go under judges who you know are sympathetic and gentle with exhibits and you will often find that once the show ring routine becomes familiar and no longer strange and threatening the problem will lessen and eventually disappear. It needs perseverence, understanding and a certain amount of firmness - and the courage to retire from the ring if the judge is being too rough with the dogs. One bad experience can set a youngster back months.

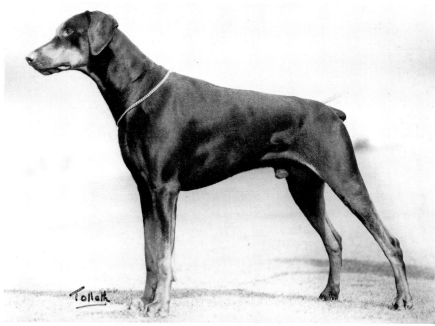

Ch Findjans Chaos. Bred and owned by Mr & Mrs Page. Winner of 6 C.C.s, 3 R.C.C.s. Top Winning Dobermann 1984. Son of the great champion Findjans Poseidon.

Ch Findjans Bo Derek of Nyewood. Bred by Mr & Mrs Page. Owned by Mrs J. Rutter.

Ch Dizown the Hustler. Bred and owned by Mrs D. Patience. Winner of 4 C.C.s, 3 R.C.C.s, J.W. A Champion at 20 months.

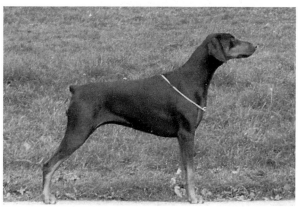

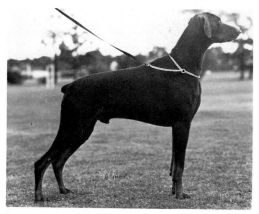

The Dobermann is a sensitive and intelligent animal and is far more aware than you probably realise of the tensions, emotions and characters around in the family situation and elsewhere. His outlook on life can be considerably altered by the surrounding situation and you will understand him better if you keep this constantly in mind. Your treatment of him and attitude to him will have an enormous influence on the way he behaves himself, and he is quite likely to be a better judge of human characters around you than you are yourself! Whatever he is, the Dobermann is no fool and most of the problems we humans have in dealing with him are of our own making.

3 Buying a Dobermann

You have now finally decided that you would like to own a Dobermann but before you dash out and buy the first puppy you see, please ask yourself the following questions.

1 Have I the time to give to a young puppy and am I patient and sympathetic?
2 Have I sufficient space indoors and out for a tiny puppy weighing only a few pounds now, to one that will grow large and weigh more than 80–90 lb (36–41 kg) in the next few months?
3 Have I enough garden to let my puppy out and is it well fenced in and dog proofed and will I mind if all my beautiful plants and flowers are dug up and my lawn spoiled?
4 Where can I exercise my dog safely away from traffic? Have I the time to take him out twice a day, in winter, in the freezing cold or on a wet and miserable day when I would sooner be by the warm fireside, or can I find the time in the early morning in summer before the day gets too hot to take him for a walk and again later in the evening before I go to bed when it is cooler?
5 Will I be able to feed my new puppy adequately now, and when he is a grown dog and eating more? Also will I be able to afford regular vaccinations and boosters to protect him from disease?
6 Can I afford vet fees in illness or in the event of an accident?
7 Is my temperament the correct temperament to manage such an intelligent dog?
8 Have I the time to feed, groom and train my new puppy and take on the obligation of making the dog part of the family for ever?
9 Am I prepared to stay at home when puppy is growing up and to give him all the time that is essential for him to grow into a calm, happy, good tempered, well balanced dog, or will I have to leave him for hours on end to make his own pleasure and become bored and destructive?
10 Is my family environment likely to change in the near future?
11 Can I make adequate arrangements for him when holidays come around?
12 Do all the family want a dog?
13 Do I really want a dog and do I really have the time?

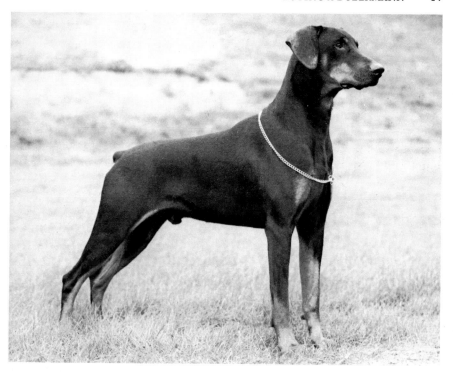

Royal Bertie of
Chevington. Bred by
R. Skinner. Owned
by O. Neave.
Winner of 3 C.C.s,
8 R.C.C.s, J.W.

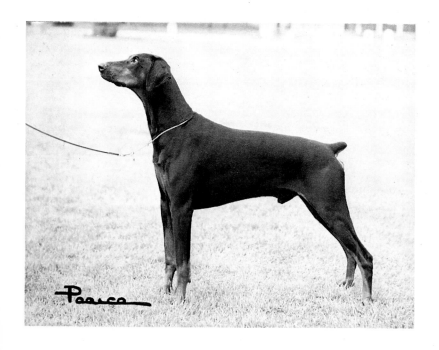

Ch Major
Marauder. Bred by
Mrs Horan. Owned
by Mr & Mrs T.
Jones. Winner of 25
C.C.s, 16 Best of
Breed. Winner of
4 Groups. Winner
of 3 Reserve Groups.
Best in Show
Welkes 1979.

Choosing a puppy and what to look for

It makes very good sense to buy a puppy near to your home. It is a comfort to know that the breeder is close at hand should you be worried about anything, especially in the early days, but don't buy close to home if you are not happy with the quality of the puppies you see. Of course if you are buying a puppy for the show ring you may well have to travel a long way to find a puppy with show potential, and even just buying a pet you could well travel to find the right quality. Naturally you will want to keep in touch with the breeder and the breeder most certainly will with you, to follow the progress of the puppy.

My advice first and foremost is to buy your puppy from a reputable breeder. If you do not know anyone who breeds Dobermanns then either contact the Kennel Club and purchase a copy of the *Kennel Gazette* (this magazine cost 60p and lists the serious breeders) or send a stamped addressed envelope to the Kennel Club for a list of breeders. You could also contact the Dog Breeders Association, an established company to which many serious breeders belong.

Visit several breeders and do take your time. Tell the breeder what you expect from your dog and they will help you to choose the right puppy for your environment and life style. Do not buy from advertisements in local or national papers, go to somebody who knows about the breed and who has many years experience. If you do this you will buy a quality puppy. Time will tell if it is a potential show specimen but your priority is to buy for temperament.

Most responsible breeders thoroughly screen buyers for their puppies and this is important both for your sake and also that of the puppy. Your own survey of the breeder's attitude, the surroundings in which the puppies are brought up and reared and the advice and friendship of the breeder who takes a continuing interest in puppies after the sale is of inestimable value to you. None of these advantages are yours if you buy from a pet shop, dealer or a puppy farmer where puppies are brought in from a number of sources. When you view the puppies try and see one or both the parents and any other dogs that they may have bred – this will help you to see what type and temperament you will be getting from this breeder.

Because of Canine Parvo Virus (a highly infectious disease in dogs to which young puppies are especially vulnerable) you could be asked to spray your shoes before entering the house and before seeing the puppies and breeders may also be wary of waking puppies as they need their sleep so always make arrangements with the breeder to visit – don't just turn up on the off chance.

If you feel something is lacking in the care or condition, look elsewhere and do not be put off if the breeder says she has many people on her waiting list, this may well be true, but if you are not happy do go away and think about it before making a decision. Never ever buy in haste.

Never buy a puppy unless he looks lively and alert with sleek skin and fat tummy and sparkling eyes. Look for a masculine dog and feminine looking bitch. Dogs are generally bigger than bitches.

When you have made your choice, leave a deposit and get a receipt and ask the breeder to mark the chosen puppy for your identification (this is usually done with nail polish on a nail or a coloured spray under puppy's arm). Return to visit the puppy at least once before you bring him home. In the meantime do try and learn all you can about your new addition to the family.

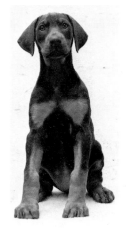

Dizown Hombre
aged 10 weeks.

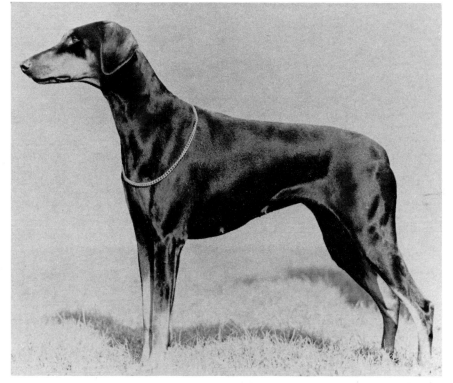

Findjans Perfecta, J.W., R.C.C. Bred and owned by Mr & Mrs Page. Dam of many of today's winners, J.W. holders and R.C.C. Winners.

I am often asked about Dobermanns with cropped ears. Cropping the ears of Dobermanns is not allowed in this country and if you do happen to have seen a dog with his ears cropped this was done before he was imported into this country. It is illegal to have ears cropped in this country and do not allow people to tell you otherwise.

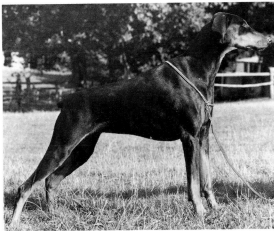

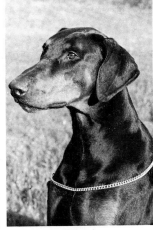

Findjans Lucrezia of Gekelven. Bred by Mr & Mrs Page. Owned by Mr & Mrs Irven.

Findjans Double Chance, J.W. Bred by Mr & Mrs Page. Owned by Mr & Mrs Meredith.

These four dogs are all from the same litter and are Ch Findjans Chaos's first sons and daughter:

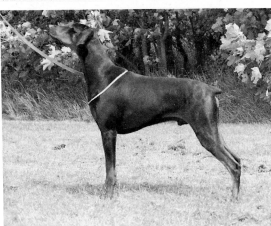

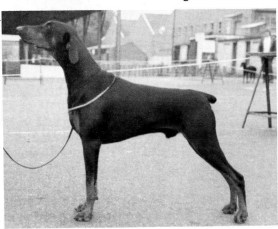

Findjans Cesare. Bred by Mr & Mrs Page. Owned by Mr & Mrs Bowring.

Findjans Giovanni of Mascoll, J.W. Bred by Mr & Mrs Page. Owned by Mrs B. Collins & Mr D. Anderson.

Another point I would like to make and that is when you buy your puppy bitch, buy her outright. Often breeders will offer a bitch puppy to a prospective buyer and offer it on breeding terms. This is not a practice to be undertaken by a newcomer to the breed. Some people are so keen to have a bitch puppy and cannot always afford one when they find out what price the puppy is and often a breeder will offer a bitch on terms.

Stay clear of this practice, it commits you to mating your bitch at some future date, to however many litters may be necessary before the breeder is satisfied. You may not be in a position to have a litter at home, your bitch may be barren and be forced to go through the traumas of being mated and unable to have puppies, and you may not have time yourself to rear a litter of puppies. It is a tremendous amount of work, hard work, and takes a lot of money to rear a litter properly. Do not commit your newly found puppy to this sort of future. There may also be problems in the blood lines that would make her a bad bet for breeding.

Before you finally take your puppy away, do ask the breeder to give you a letter stating that if you cannot for any reason keep your puppy at a later date, she will definitely take the puppy back herself. If you have gone to a breeder who cares this should not present a problem as I know that the majority of breeders take this precaution already. As a matter of routine they follow the progress of each puppy sold, and they encourage the purchaser to keep in touch. If a breeder is reluctant to give you this assurance then I would ask you to look elsewhere. It will be hard, but if everyone followed a code of ethics the breed would become better protected and preserved – which is after all what we would all like to see.

There are four colours in the Breed Standard – Black, Brown, Blue and Isabella – and there should be no price difference between any of them. No colour is rare so don't be fooled by being told otherwise.

Male or female?

This is a personal choice. Some people want a dog because they cannot be bothered with a bitch having seasons, others prefer bitches and others don't seem to mind which they have. The important thing to remember is that if you have a bitch she needs greater care. She must not be mated before she is two years old and when she is in season, which lasts roughly three weeks, needs to be protected all the time.

Never, ever, buy two dogs or two bitches from any one litter. Until you have gone through all the stages of your first puppy it is better to leave a second purchase until your puppy is well over a year old. They have very boisterous teenage years, anything from ten to fourteen months and sometimes at this stage you are wondering how on earth you will cope, and what on earth you have bought.

Do not allow your dog to be used as a stud and it should always be under control in the company of a female dog in season. It is a great mistake to allow your pet dog to mate a pet bitch of someone you know, stud work is best left to the professionals, as faulty puppies can occur if the pedigrees of the parents do not match. Should however an accident occur and you find your dog mating a bitch (they start very young and when you least expect it,) do not panic. Many novice people have never seen dogs mate and they cannot understand when they see a dog and a bitch back to back. Do not try and prise them apart because you will damage both the dog and the bitch. Do not attempt to throw water over them either, if it has happened just let it take its natural course, they will separate when the act is over. Take your bitch along to the vet straight away for an injection, because there is nothing worse than an unwanted litter, and these always seem to be to the worse possible combinations of dogs.

Puppy or adult?

Whilst you might feel that giving an older dog a home might be easier than perhaps having a young puppy, it is important to bear in mind that sometimes dogs looking for a second or third home may have some behavioural problem, which is why they are now unwanted by their previous owners and you may not find out what the problem is until something drastic happens. It is therefore very important to find out the background of the dog before contemplating rehousing it. Dobermann Rescue go to great lengths to find out the history of every dog before placing that dog in a suitable home, so it is wise to approach them rather than take a dog off someone you do not know.

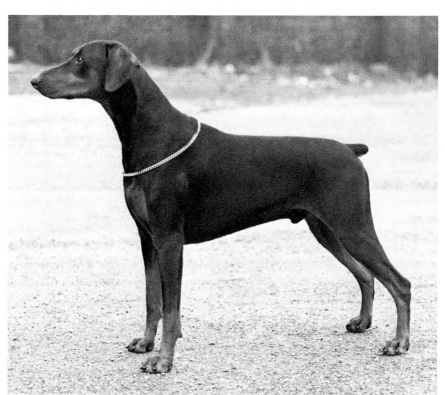

Ch Chornytan Fable. Bred by Mrs Thelma Toole. Owned by Mr Gandley. Winner of 9 C.C.s, 11 R.C.C.s.

Alternatively you may be fortunate in taking on someone's well loved pet who sadly cannot be kept for some genuine reason. Most dogs will respond to love and kindness but especially if you have children be particularly careful in taking on an older dog from someone who just doesn't want him anymore.

In taking on an adult dog it is important not to leave it alone for any length of time until you thoroughly understand the way it reacts and until the dog feels secure in its new home. Newly acquired dogs are easily lost when off the lead and become disorientated because they are trying to find their own home and owner. Even if the dog is good and comes when called in the garden, do not rely on your control over it outside the home until two or three months have passed.

Points to look for

1 A clean environment, whether puppies are in a run outside and in an outdoor kennel, or kept inside the house, everywhere should be clean and unsoiled.
2 The puppy should look strong and healthy and have a pliant skin like a seal and dark sparkling almond shaped eyes with an alert expression. He should have good round bone and strong hind-quarters, good top-line, long arched neck and good clean cut head with blunt muzzle, small ears and good rich rust markings. He should be friendly and not cower at the sight of strangers (cowering could indicate nervousness).
3 Puppies' tails should be nice and clean and healthy looking. Many puppies are sold with badly docked tails which have to be re-docked again at six months. This is a traumatic experience and a painful and worrying time for the puppy up until that age, also it is quite dangerous as an extremely badly docked tail can lead to many serious problems, if neglected.
4 When choosing your puppy, try and choose one from a litter where both parents are certified free of HD & CVI (*see* Glossary).
5 Never bring a puppy home earlier than seven or eight weeks.
6 Ensure the mouth is correct i.e. when teeth (front) just overlap bottom front teeth.

What to avoid

1 Puppies with dull or runny eyes.
2 Puppies with a cough or diarrhoea and which are listless.

3   Skin with red blotches – if these are present this could indicate mange, ringworm, eczema or fungus.
4   Crooked legs as these could mean rickets and they should not be potbellied.

Checklist before bringing puppy home

1   Decide the areas in your home your puppy is to use and parts of the garden that will be his. Make a run in the garden which can easily be erected for the puppy to go in for his rest and play during the day, while you get on with your chores and make this his place of refuge where he can go when he wants to be alone.
2   Check fences and gates and ensure they are securely latched and that they are out of reach of young children who might inadvertently leave a gate open.
3   Reposition all trailing electricity leads and telephone wires, which the puppy may find and chew.
4   Cover sandpits, deep ponds and swimming pools.
5   Remove household and garden chemicals especially poisonous slug pellets which are so dangerous and often fatal to dogs, to absolutely safe storage.
6   Explain to the children the dangers of leaving their small plastic toys around. Keep tights and stockings and other nylon underwear out of puppy's reach as these are the cause of many emergency operations and if not treated in time can kill your puppy if he has swallowed them without your realising it.
7   Any toys, bones or bowls should not be left out over night for fear of soiling by mice and rats which might risk your puppy catching leptospirosis.
8   Arrange front door drill with your family and make sure everyone knows it. Puppies can dart quickly through your legs when answering the door and be out on the road and killed or the cause of an accident before you realise it.

Pedigrees, forms and registration papers

Even though you have set about buying your Dobermann the right way (by going to a reputable and well established breeder) you must still be fully aware of the problems which can occur when obtaining a pedigree.

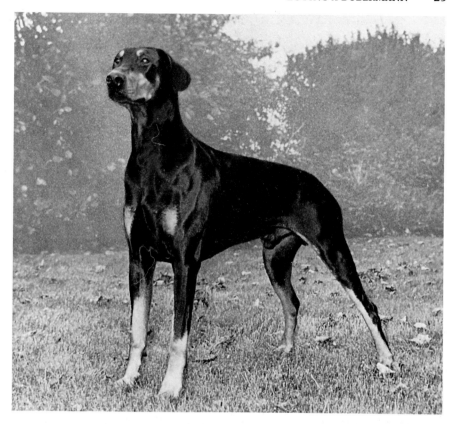

Ch Davalogs
Crusader. Owned by
Mr & Mrs Alan
Mulholland.

Unfortunately there are a number of people who give false pedigrees and because the buyer of the puppy is often unaware of the procedure I have listed below the various points you must look for, when you are collecting your puppy and all the bits and pieces the breeder must give with the puppy. On the following pages I have shown a pedigree and highlighted what should be on the pedigree of your dog. I have also shown examples of the transfer forms and the registration forms you should be given to complete and which will be returned by the Kennel Club.

You may have seen the pedigree of the parents of your puppy when you first went along to choose him, so you will have a good idea from that and will notice familiar names on your own puppy's pedigree. Make certain everything ties up with the colour, sex and age of the puppy on the form and that you haven't got a black bitch puppy on the form and that you are taking home a brown dog puppy.

When you collect your puppy, you will most likely have paid a small deposit and naturally you take this amount off the price. If you are paying cash make absolutely certain you get a receipt for the money, if you pay by cheque your cheque stub is usually good enough as a receipt.

The breeder may have registered the puppies as a litter and in that case you will receive a form (see(1)) and this you will need to send to the Kennel Club Registrations Department with the required fee. The breeder may have registered the puppy as an individual and therefore the puppy will be named, but you will need to send the form to the Kennel Club and you will also need to ask for a Change of Ownership form and for the puppy to go on the Active Register.

Transfer forms may occasionally be late due to the original names chosen by the breeder not being accepted by the Kennel Club and therefore the breeder has to reapply for new names which takes time and may not be in the breeder's hands until after you have collected your puppy. It is very important that the breeder has also signed the Transfer form.

THE KENNEL CLUB

Registration Certificate for: FINDJANS LUCREZIA H10

Registration No. H3941001H10

Breed	DOBERMANN	Sex BITCH	Born 20/04/83	Registered 18/07/83
Colour	BLACK	Breeder MR M G & MRS A J PAGE
Sire	FINDJANS CHAOS G11 G4163705G11
Dam	FINDJANS PERFECTA F10 2829BR

TRANSFERRED ON 30/07/83 FROM MR M G AND MRS A J PAGE

Owned by   MR & MRS G IRVEN
                 'FOXLANDS'
                 24 BRACKENDALE CLOSE CAMBERLEY
                 SURREY GU15 1HP

                                                    23/08/83   01/09/83

The issue of this certificate does not guarantee its accuracy as it is based on details supplied to The Kennel Club by the applicant. The code which follows the name of a dog indicates the month and year of the issue of the KCSB Breed Records Supplement in which the notice of the registration appears.

SAMPLE

APPLICATION TO REGISTER A TRANSFER

FROM Mr / Mrs / Miss _____

Address _____

_____

Signature(s) (see Note 3) _____

Date of Transfer of Ownership _____
IMPORTANT If the dog named overleaf has been entered for any shows or trials by the previous owner and the new owner has purchased the dog with these engagements, the following undertaking must be signed by the new owner(s).

I/We undertake to abide by the conditions of entry made by Mr / Mrs / Miss _____

_____ on _____

at the_____ shows/trials

Signature of Owner(s)_____
1. Please write in ink. Use BLOCK CAPITALS for all names with the exception of the signatures to the declaration.
2. An application will not be accepted if any alterations or deletions are made to the names of the previous or present owners.
3. If for any reason the previous owner's signature cannot be obtained, application for for transfer can be made to the Committee on this form supported by an explanation, purchase receipt and any other relevant documents.
4. The declaration must be signed by all the owners in the case of a joint ownership.
5. When submitted this form remains the property of the Kennel Club.

TO Mr / Mrs / Miss _____

Address _____

_____

_____

I/We have read the instructions for the completion of this form and agree to be bound and submit to Kennel Club Rules and Regulations as the same may be amended from time to time.

Date_____ Signature(s)_____

FOR OFFICIAL USE ONLY

SAMPLE

FEE SEE LIST OF FEES
    As published in The Kennel Gazette
If you require a VAT invoice, please initial the box →

8/11/81   © The Kennel Club

On the pedigree you will need to look for the Kennel Club Registration Number, date of registration and make sure the breeder has completed their name and address and do check that these are the same as the address you are collecting the puppy from.

BREED: DOBERMANN **SEX:** BITCH **COLOUR & MARKINGS:** BLACK & TAN **DATE OF BIRTH:** 20th April 1983 **NAME:** FINDJANS LUCREZIA OF GEKELVEN **PET NAME:** SOPHIE	**P E D I G R E E**		**REGISTRATION NO.** H394100 H 10 **REGISTRATION DATE:** 15th July 1983 **OWNER:** MR & MRS G IRVEN FOXLANDS 24 BRACKENDALE CLOSE CAMBERLEY SURREY
PARENTS	**GRAND-PARENTS**	**GREAT GRAND-PARENTS**	**G.G.GRAND-PARENTS**
Sire: CH.FINDJANS CHAOS Name & Address of Owner: Mr & Mrs M Page 35 Ruskin Road Chadwell St.Mary Grays. Essex.	Sire: CH.FINDJANS POSEIDON Dam: Findjans Atropos	Sire: Phileens Duty Free of Tavey Dam: CH.MITRASANDRA GAY LADY OF FINDJANS Sire: CH.ARKTURUS VALANS CHOICE Dam: CH.MITRASANDRA GAY LADY OF FINDJANS	Sire:AM.CH.TARRODOS CORRY Dam: Kayhills Outrigger Sire:CH.TUMLOW SATAN Dam: Findjans Fair Allyne Sire: Linhoff The Pagan Dam:Findjans Princess Pleasurance Sire: CH.TUMLOW SATAN Dam: Findjans Fair Allyne
Dam: Findjans Perfecta Name & Address of Owner Mr & Mrs M Page 35 Ruskin Road Chadwell St.Mary Grays. Essex.	Sire: CH.DAVALOGS CRUSADER Dam: CH.FINDJANS FREYA	Sire: CH.TUMLOW SATAN Dam: Edwina Vivacious Sire: CH.FINDJANS POSEIDON Dam: Tanerdyce Michealia	Sire: CH.TUMLOW IMPECCABLE Dam: Tumlow Odette Sire: Nvrilla Gay Crusader Dam: Tumlow Vivacious Sire:Phileens Duty Free of Tavey Dam:CH.MITRASANDRA GAY LADY OF FINDJANS Sire:CH.HEIDILAND TROUBLE SPOT Dam: Ashendens Primo Tullah
BREEDER: MR & MRS M PAGE 35 RUSKIN ROAD CHADWELL ST MARY GRAYS. ESSEX.		I /WE CERTIFY THAT THE ABOVE PARTICULARS ARE CORRECT..................	

Checklist of supplies required before bringing puppy home

1 Supply of food in accordance with breeder's diet sheet (which they will have discussed with you on an earlier visit).
2 Liquid paraffin and special kaolin mixture as made up for babies from your chemist.
3 Waterbowl and food dish.
4 Hide chews (not those from Taiwan or South Korea as they contain a substance which can make dogs very ill). A large marrow bone.
5 Disinfectant for floors and 'No Stain' for carpets.
6 A mild disinfectant like Dettol or Formula H correctly diluted for everything in contact with the puppy.
7 Bed (plastic baskets are easy to wipe clean and more hygienic).
8 Bedding – vetbed or blankets.
9 Tools for picking up excreta in the garden (or install a doggy loo).
10 Puppy collar and lead.
11 Vet's telephone number and that of the breeder by the telephone.
12 Hot water bottle and cover and ticking clock for puppy's first few nights.

Safeguarding your puppy

INSURANCE

Insuring your puppy is not only a sensible and realistic line to take but a reassurance for you that should your puppy become ill you can meet the veterinary bills without the worry of trying to find the money and most importantly that you can take the puppy to the vet for immediate attention and care and not be embarrassed about running up a large bill.

There are several good organisations that deal with pet insurance and these I list below:

Pet Plan Ltd.,
319–327 Chiswick High Road,
London W4 4HH
Telephone (01)995–5281

Private Pet Policies (Vetwise),
Orient House,
42/5 New Broadstreet,
London EC2 M1QY
Telephone (01)-628-0305

Dog Breeders Insurance Co. Ltd.,
12 Christchurch Road,
Lansdowne,
Bournemouth BH1 3LE
Telephone (0202)295771

Your vet most likely will operate a scheme and it is to your advantage and peace of mind to take advantage of one or other of these schemes.

DOG LICENCE

A dog licence is necessary for your dog at 6 months of age and is renewable every year. This is obtainable from the Post Office and at the time of writing this book costs 37p.

TATTOOING

Another very sound way of protecting your pet is by tattooing. This is a harmless method and painless for the dog. Your National Insurance Number is tattooed on the inside of the dog's right hind leg and then should your dog ever be lost, he can always be brought back to you as all the police stations and animal hostels are now familiar with this procedure. For information contact either:

The Central Dog Registry,
49 Marlowes Road,
London W8 6LA

or

Mrs A. Stone,
56 Albion Road,
Hounslow,
Middlesex,
Telephone 01 572 7848

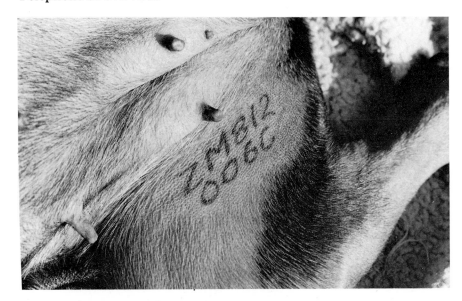

Dobermann showing her tattoo which is a sound way of protecting your pet should it ever be lost. All police stations and animal hostels are now familiar with this procedure.

The RSPCA also have a scheme whereby cards are given to be carried and in the event of an accident or illness or suddenly being admitted to hospital the person nominated to care for your pet is contacted. These cards and information on this scheme are obtainable from:
RSPCA
The Causeway,
Horsham,
Sussex.
(Please send a SAE when making enquiries.)

4   Caring for the puppy

Bringing your new puppy home

Bringing your new puppy home is such an exciting event and arrangements to collect your new addition to the family should be made when all the family are home and nothing else important is happening. Assuming you will collect your puppy in a car, take someone along with you who is willing to hold the puppy on the journey home as this will make him feel more secure – take a couple of towels and an old jumper or cardigan to wrap round him for extra cosiness. It is worth remembering that an uncontrollable puppy as large as an eight week old Dobermann can make driving a hazard and positively dangerous if there is no one to hold him.

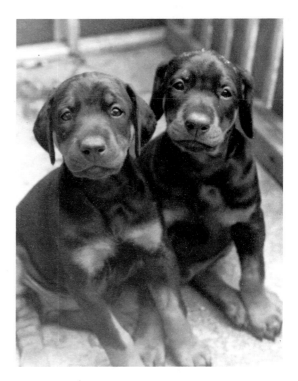

An adorable pair of Dobermann puppies.

On your way home, talk to the puppy and do remember not to let him out of the car on the journey. It is best to go straight home, and settle your puppy in as soon as possible. On arrival feed him with warm milk and let him get to know you. Let him wander around, he will be feeling very strange and lonely and missing his mother and his litter brothers and sisters.

Now that you actually have your beautiful, appealing Dobermann puppy with soft eyes and plump belly and oversized legs and feet, home at last, let him find out about you, let him wander around and find his smells, when he comes to you let him sniff his fill, scratch him behind the ears and pat him, then ignore him for a little while. Teach your children the correct way to hold your Dobermann puppy. Never pick him up by the scruff of his neck, always lift the puppy gently with both hands and with one hand under the chest and thumbs over the elbows and the other hand supporting his hindquarters. Take care not to poke a finger in his soft tummy. It is better not to let young children pick up the puppy at all whilst he is very young for fear of dropping him.

He will probably be missing his litter mates and will most likely cry the first night or two, so wrap a hot water bottle in a blanket or towel and put these under his blanket. Wrap a ticking clock up too, this will remind him of his mother's heart and put that in his bed for added comfort. Take the trouble to settle him properly the first night and you will soon have trouble-free uninterrupted sleep yourself.

Check list on collecting your puppy from the breeder

1 Diet sheet.
2 Worming certificate.
3 Vaccination/innoculation certificate* (which you should give to your vet when you take your puppy for a check-up and he will advise you on the ages he will want to vaccinate the puppy).
4 Pedigree of puppy.
5 Registration form 2 which you send off to the Kennel Club.

*Do remember to make an appointment with your vet before you collect the puppy, don't just turn up unannounced. Many vets do not vaccinate puppies until they are eight weeks at least and more likely twelve weeks so do not be surprised if you do not get a vaccination certificate. Some breeders may give a parvo injection before selling any of their stock and you should take this card to your vet who will decide when to fully vaccinate your puppy.

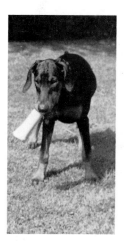

Puppy 'Look what I've found'.

Minor ailments

Having a puppy in the home is like having a new baby around and it is not always easy to distinguish serious problems from minor ailments which affect most puppies during the growing up period.

As with all young animals, puppies are up and down very rapidly. By the time you have phoned your vet the pain and the symptoms may well have gone. Nevertheless, early diagnosis and treatment can save your puppy a lot of trouble. So as a brief guide here are some of the minor ailments which your puppy is likely to experience.

1   Puppies tend to chew everything they can find: they will eat coal and dirt and will likely vomit them up again. A toy or a dog chew will help to keep them amused. They usually grow out of these habits but if the puppy continues to eat coal or dirt, see your vet. Puppies are often indiscriminate eaters and therefore their motions may vary in colour and consistency, they will be softer, lighter and less well formed, puppies also pass motions much more frequently than an adult dog. Any signs of prolonged diarrhoea, spots of blood or loss of body weight should be reported to your vet.
2   Puppies should be active and respond to you and your family but they do need to sleep a lot. If your puppy doesn't show a reasonable amount of activity and alertness between periods of rest he should be checked out by a vet.
3   The most obvious signs of health and ill health are seen in the eyes, the skin and the mouth. Puppies' eyes should be clear and bright. The skin and coat should be bright, shiny and supple. The colour inside the mouth should be pale pink.
4   Puppies have temporary and permanent teeth. The milk teeth are usually shed between 4 and 6 months.
5   Most puppies scratch themselves on and off during the day, any continual scratching and obvious loss of hair and inflammation of skin should be reported to your vet.

General Notes On Care

1   Do not change the puppy's diet too drastically. I have always fed my puppies on finely minced black or green tripe and puppy meal twice a day with cereal and scrambled eggs for two milk feeds (see diet sheet). Never change the brand of milk suddenly and never feed tinned dog food, unless it is one specially formulated for young puppies.

2   Your puppy needs and must have lots of sleep and the children should not be allowed to pull him around.

3   With a young puppy around watchfulness and anticipation are key words. Do not allow him to climb up or down stairs until he is very much older. If you have other dogs do not allow them to play with the puppy while he is so young, keep an ever watchful eye on them in the garden. Puppies' bones break easily and accidents happen so quickly.

4   Children and dogs should be trained to behave perfectly with each other and children must be taught to respect a Dobermann as they are a breed of dog which does not tolerate being teased.

5   Do not show your puppy off to all the family, friends and neighbours immediately. He is so young and has only just left his family and everything will be strange to him. Take things gently, there is plenty of time to show him off later.

6   You have now brought your puppy home, it is a very exciting occasion for you and the family but a traumatic one for your little fellow who has just left his mother and brothers and sisters and is now facing the big wide world alone with you. Follow your breeder's instructions implicitly, talk to the puppy quietly and reassuringly and if you leave him make sure you leave him in a safe place where no danger can come to him.

7   You can buy a proper dog cage, and put him in that as a sort of indoor kennel which will keep him out of harm while you nip to the shops etc. and he will get used to it and go in there of his own accord when he wants to go to sleep.

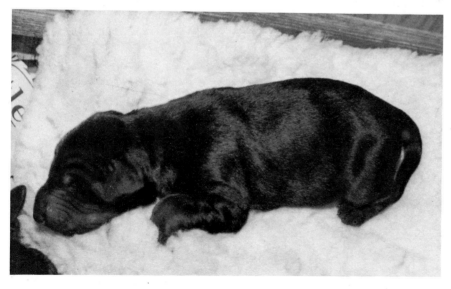

Puppy 3 days old.

8 Within twenty-four hours of bringing your puppy home take him to your vet for a check up. Usually the breeder will ask you to do this anyway and if there is anything wrong the breeder will normally take the puppy back.

9 Nowadays as vets' fees are so high it is prudent to have some form of insurance to cover vet bills. Apart from being a wise and practical decision to take this gives you peace of mind knowing that your puppy in the event of an accident or illness is protected in more ways than one and you have peace of mind knowing the bills will be met.

Puppy's bed and toys

Decide where your puppy is to sleep and keep its bed there. The bed should be either a cardboard box lined with a blanket while it is very small or a hard plastic bed which is really best as it can be wiped out daily.

For the first two weeks you may need to keep the puppy beside you when you sleep as puppies left on their own straight away cry and get hysterical – it is better for you and puppy to be close until your puppy gets its bearings. Remember companionship, touch and comfort are KEYWORDS.

Give puppy chews and hide bones but not those from South Korea or Asia as some of them contain a poisonous substance which makes dogs ill. Large marrow bones, rubber balls and hardwood logs are all lovely toys for your new little friend. Do not give old shoes or old clothes as dogs cannot distinguish between old and new – believe me I have learned this from experience.

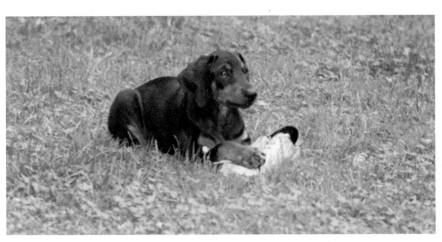

Puppy with master's shoe.

Do make sure that puppy's bed and where it is kept are sufficiently ventilated as there have been an increasing number of cases reported of dogs being poisoned from the fumes of solid fuel boilers.

Never ever leave things like tights, or pop socks lying around as these are most dangerous to an inquisitive puppy, as indeed they are to a grown dog, and if swallowed often necessitate an operation for removal. Never leave lavatory seats up especially if bleach has just been put down, puppies are so inquisitive, and if they find themselves in the bathroom and the loo they reach down and drink the water! Never leave washing soaking in bleach within reach either.

Female puppy

Your bitch puppy may come into season any time after six months (in some extreme cases this can occur earlier even than that). When this happens she will feel strange and if anything like my young bitches will wonder what is happening to her. They run round trying to lick their rear ends, scooting on the floor and generally have a worried look about them.

Treat them gently and when the season does start you will notice her keeping herself clean. Take all the necessary precautions of making sure she is not mated early. Her temperament may change a little bit, but generally they take it all in their stride.

Make sure her bed and bedding are kept nice and fresh and clean and do not scold her if she stains the carpets. There is a very good carpet stain remover on the market and it is worthwhile having this around, and also I usually put my bitches in Petnix – these are little knickers – but do remember that when they need to go out to spend a penny or whatever, do remove them.

Never have a young bitch spayed until after her first season as this prohibits natural growth.

Male puppy

The young male puppy often differs greatly and is more difficult to handle than a bitch. The dog puppy will not fully mature until he is eighteen months to two years old and vandalism is as natural to a Dobermann as it is to boys in their teens.

From nine to eighteen months your boy Dobermann is a teenager. He may not appear to want to guard the house and many new owners are often disappointed at this apparent lack of Dobermannishness, but there always comes a time when he feels his feet as a true male.

Many people have rung up the breeder of their puppy with the plea 'how can I stop my puppy biting me', and have even gone to the extent of tying him up in the garden or beating him into 'submission' telling everyone that he is a vicious animal, when in fact he is probably just teething.

Your puppy may be a mild fellow, on the other hand he could be full of fire, needing a firm but kind hand to help him adjust to your household.

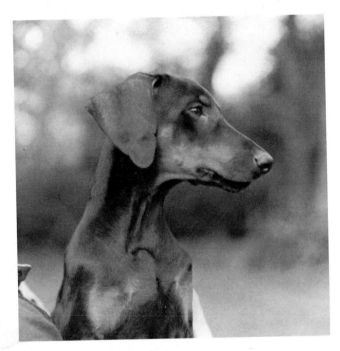

A lovely headstudy of Findjans Hassle, 14 weeks. Bred by Mr & Mrs Page. Owned by Mrs Page & Mrs Irven.

Feeding your Puppy

DIET PLAN

The following diet plan is suggested, but you can vary the amount of biscuit, meat and milk either way to suit your own particular Dobermann puppy's requirement. If the puppy seems very hungry then do increase the food but do not over feed or give titbits in between meals. Some puppies need more food than I have suggested to reach their full potential. The main ingredients are meat, biscuit, milk, eggs and cereal but there are a few commercially prepared puppy foods on the market which are completely satisfactory.

A general vitamin-mineral supplement and a specific calcium supplement should be given; I always give Canovel Vitamin/Mineral Tablets and Canovel Calcium Tablets, there are of course other makes available. Provided these are given as recommended and the diet is adequate there should be no need for further supplementation.

If ever you are in doubt ask your vet's advice and stick to it and always read the manufacturer's instructions very carefully and adhere to them strictly.

A puppy requiring strong heavy bone should have calcium added to his diet (this is given in the Calcium tablets suggested above). Do not go mad and think the more calcium the more bone. Too much added vitamins could prove harmful.

8 to 12 weeks	*5 meals a day*
Breakfast	½ pint warm milk
	1 tablespoon Farex/Readybreak
Lunch	4 oz (113 g) minced beef and 2 oz (56 g) puppy meal (increase meat by 2 oz (56 g) weekly to 8 oz (226 g) at 12 weeks)
	Biscuit should be increased in proportion each week.
	For a change, white fish, or scrambled egg or minced chicken can be given instead of minced beef, with the puppy biscuit meal.
Tea	½ pint (·28 l) warm milk with a beaten-up egg
Supper	Same as lunch
Nightcap	warm milk

During this period the puppy will start teething and the intake of calcium should be increased. Flying ears and slack feet are often an indication of insufficient calcium, but do read manufacturers instructions carefully.

13 to 16 weeks	4 meals a day
	Drop the 4 pm feed and change from beef to tripe.
17 to 24 weeks	4 meals a day
	Drop midday feed
6 months to 12 months	3 meals a day
	2 meat and one milk feed
12 months onwards	2 meals a day
Breakfast	milk with biscuit and egg
Dinner	1 lb (·45 kg) meat 6 oz (168 g) biscuit

As an alternative you may like to use Pedigree Chum Puppy Food which has been formulated following years of successful investigations by Pedigree Petfoods Animal Studies Centre Europe's foremost authority on petcare and nutrition.

It is designed to be fed either by itself or with a biscuit such as Pedigree Chum Mixer or puppy meal on the basis of three volumes Pedigree Chum Puppy Food to two volumes of biscuits. From about four months the quantity of biscuit can be increased to equal volumes of puppy food and biscuit.

For puppies less than three months old it is advisable to soften the biscuit with hot milk or water ten minutes prior to feeding. Older puppies seem to enjoy crunching the biscuit. The quantities of food that a puppy needs vary enormously depending on the age and the character of the particular puppy.

The condition of your puppy is the best indicator of whether you are feeding the correct amount. Generally a puppy should be given as much as he will eat in fifteen minutes at each meal. After fifteen minutes leftover food should be removed and fresh food served at the next meal. Remember to ensure your puppy always has fresh drinking water available to him.

House training

Puppies should be restricted in the house whilst very young so that should an awkward accident occur, it can be seen. In puppies, as in babies, feeding and elimination follow each other very quickly so you must be ready to take your puppy outside the instant it has finished eating. Also immediately the puppy wakens you will need to be ready. Agitation and being left alone and crying will make puppy pass urine.

You will notice that during play the puppy will sniff around the floor in a tight circle, looking worried when it has the urge to go, but the interval between indication and doing it is very short. The time between indication and elimination gets longer and the older the puppy the clearer the signal will be given, progressing to actually asking. All our Dobermanns tap on the door when they want to go out.

The word you use for housetraining must be decided when you first get the puppy and it must then be used every time the act is performed in the right place. We always use the word 'bibis' and when the puppy is sniffing around the garden last thing at night or early morning with you saying bibis you do feel a bit like a raving lunatic, but it does work eventually! Praise puppy when they do go.

It takes a lot of patience as the puppy's concentration wanders when it is outside and sees the butterflies and birds etc and he forgets what he has gone out there for. At other times, during bad weather especially, put newspaper by the door and move the newspaper outside as the weather improves. It might be worth noting that if the first puddle of the day is done out in the garden the puppy will become clean very quickly (so set your alarm very early!)

Chewing

All puppies chew, every puppy goes through this teething process and can be very destructive if not carefully watched. When a puppy picks up an object to chew, remove it from him with a sharp 'NO' and replace it with a toy.

Remember to close all cupboard and wardrobe doors as puppies are dab hands at finding your best shoes. I learnt to close all doors and put away anything of value very early on after spending a fortune on replacing shoes and gloves. Cushions, pillows, quilts and comforters are all a puppy's delight, so be on your guard, play safe, and keep your puppy confined to his own quarters if you are busy and cannot watch what he is up to.

Do watch houseplants carefully. Many times I have turned my back and have been busy in the house, only to find headless plants all over the place, and spotted the puppy haring round with a plant in her mouth, shaking hell out of it, dirt flying all over the carpet, leaves scattered everywhere. I love my puppies but I also love my houseplants, so a word of advice is keep everything that you value well out of reach.

Exercising your puppy

Puppies do not need a lot of exercise and certainly cannot be taken out until after the last vaccination. You should then start with gentle road walks. I never free run any of my puppies until they are nine to ten months old. They have a large garden in which to play and have fifteen to twenty minutes road walking morning and night. As they get older I take them somewhere safe to free run (titbit in pocket to catch them first time they are off the lead!)

Take your puppy out and about with you as often as you can to get them used to every possible situation. Take him to the shops and around the town and you will be surprised how many people will stop and stroke him. All this contact with people will help to make your puppy sensible, unafraid and confident. ·

5 Care of the Adult Dog

Basically it is just good common sense looking after your Dobermann and this section is written for the owners whose Dobermanns have outgrown the boisterous puppy stage and are maturing into good sensible dogs. So long as you exercise your dog adequately, train him to a reasonably acceptable standard, i.e. not to jump up at people and to walk to heel and to obey basic commands, you will have a much more enjoyable life with your dog.

An older dog really only needs one meal a day but we always feed ours breakfast and dinner. They are always exercised very early in the morning and come back from this exercise, like we do, looking forward to a snack so they all have milk and biscuits for breakfast and then their main meal in the evening.

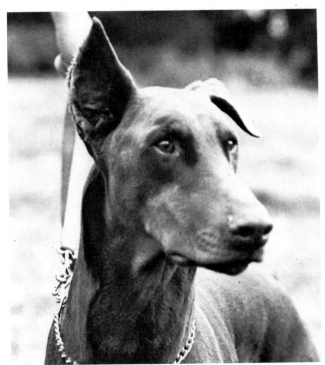

Cameron's Snoopy of Tinkazen – a Canadian import. Owned by Jean Scheja. Originally bought by a Lt Commander in the British Navy in Nova Scotia as a fully trained guard dog. Came to England and 2 days after coming out of quarantine he went to Mrs Scheja. Sire of 2 Champions.

If possible take your Dobermann out with you as often as possible as they really do thrive on companionship and with good discipline can be a real pleasure and such good company too.

Make sure you look at ears and eyes regularly, removing the jelly-like substance which appears in the corners of the eyes with a tissue, clean the ears gently, Dobes absolutely adore their ears being cleaned and grunt with sheer pleasure. Check teeth are not hurting them, you should notice if they have difficulty in eating their food, and if you suspect something is wrong take them to the vet straight away, you know how toothache hurts you, don't allow the dogs to suffer any longer than need be. Trim his nails once a week and treat him gently if he appears off colour. If he has any sickness or diarrhoea see a vet if it continues for more than twenty-four hours.

Once a year take him for his booster injections. Keep a note in your diary for this, but usually a vet will send you a reminder.

Feeding

After your puppy is a year old one meal a day is usually sufficient but as I have said we usually feed our dogs milk and biscuits after their early morning run and give them their dinner at night. Tripe (black) and wholemeal biscuits are what all my dogs are fed on and they have thrived on this. Most dogs will eat tripe.

Tinned food is all right for an emergency if you have forgotten to get tripe out of the freezer and it hasn't defrosted in time. I always defrost the tripe in large plastic containers with lids on, then one doesn't have the awful smell lingering around.

There are other foods such as tribeef, plus the brawns and complete foods. Once you have found a food which your dog will eat try and keep him on it, by giving him too much variety you will make him finicky and difficult to feed. Give your dog a change now and then, but basically keep him on the same diet unless he is ill or if he has a problem and needs a different type, your vet will advise you on this. Always have plenty of fresh drinking water around. They also love marrow bones and will spend hours gnawing away at them.

Do not feed your dog vast amounts of liver or offal, for obvious reasons this will give him violent diarrhoea.

Grooming and general care

Dobermanns generally do not need much attention to their coats if they are in good healthy condition, but your puppy must always be rubbed down and dried with a towel if he has been out in the rain. A

FIG.1

FIG.2

FIG.3

bath is not necessary unless the puppy is very dirty and then only ever on a warm day.

A Dobermann can suffer from scurf around the area where his collar fits. Unless it is very bad it is something which can be treated using a good quality shampoo or a dessert spoon of cooking oil in his food. Witch Hazel is very effective if you wipe it around the area, but this is a problem which is common to most Dobermanns.

EARS   Check once or twice a week.
Wipe carefully with dry cotton wool to remove dust, grass seeds etc.
Don't poke too deeply or use a cleaning bud or anything hard. Any dark, smelly secretion (popularly called 'Canker') should be wiped away using cotton wool and an oil based cleaner such as veterinary eardrops which is formulated to clear infection and mites and should be used as directed.

EYES   Eyes are deepset and mucus gathers in the corners. Remove this carefully with tissue or cottonwool, using a separate piece for each eye. If mucus is yellow rather than grey wipe with Optrex, if eye is red, swollen itching or painful see a vet.

NAILS   Cut nails once a week with a proper pair of nail clippers or file.

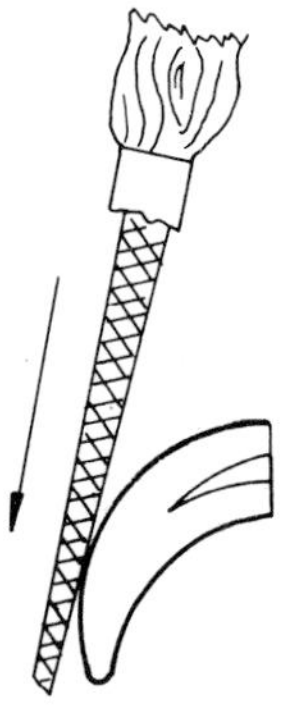

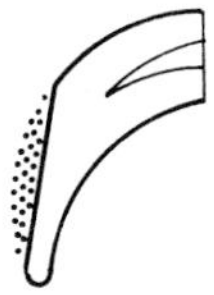

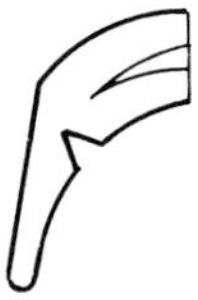

Nail Trimming Illustrated. The method illustrated is to take a sharp file and stroke the file downwards in the direction of the arrow as in Fig. 1 until it assumes the shape in Fig. 2, the shaded portion being the part removed. A three cornered file should then be used on the underside, as in Fig. 3 and the operation is then complete. The dog running about quickly wears the nail to the proper shape.

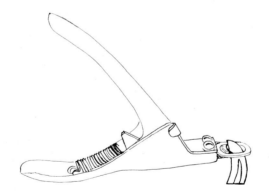

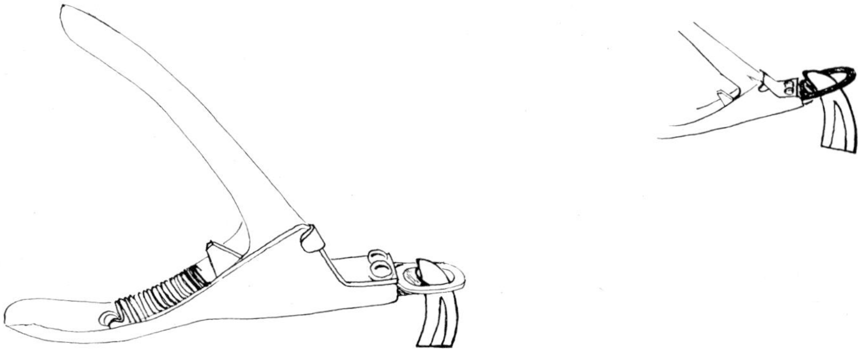

Clipping Nails Illustrated. The guillotine type clippers are the safest and easiest to use. Nails should be trimmed each week. Only the tips of nails should be clipped to begin with as it is easy to nick the vein (quick) which runs inside the nail and cause bleeding. In some breeds the vein can be seen through the nail but in the Dobermann with black nails it is not visible. If you make a mistake, bleeding can be stopped immediately by the application of a pinch of potassium permanganate or a dampened syptic pencil as used for shaving cuts.

FEET Examine regularly for cracked pads, small cuts, splinters and thorns. Examine feet daily for grass seeds. A Dobermann sometimes suffers from cysts between the toes which can become swollen and infected if left unnoticed.

TEETH Clean teeth with a brush and regular toothpaste. Have teeth scaled regularly by your vet.

Bathing

Bathing is seldom necessary, once or twice a year should be adequate but should the dog become exceptionally dirty or begin to have a nasty odour, then you will have to give him an extra bath.

First put a nylon collar and lead on your dog (leather spoils when soaked with water). If possible, tie the lead to a secure fixing, leaving both hands free. Start at the head, holding it firmly by the muzzle, face towards you, tilt the chin up. Wet the head from behind the eyes, using a spray from a mixer tap, shower unit or hose pipe connected to mixer tap if you are bathing the dog in the garden.

Hold the nozzle of the spray in your hand allowing the jets of water to pass over your fingers. This will enable you to have a continuous check on the water temperature. The closer you hold the nozzle to the dog's head, the less noise it makes, and the less frightened your Dobermann will be.

When you have thoroughly wetted the fur apply a small amount of shampoo to the top of the head, still holding the chin well up, to prevent soap running into the eyes, and lather up. If it is necessary to wash the muzzle, use a little water, and one finger dipped in shampoo. Still holding the head back, rinse off away from the eyes, then let the head drop. Allow the water to run down the face. Rinse the muzzle, do not get water in the ears.

Once the head is finished the worst is over. You then wet body, back, chest, legs, underparts etc applying shampoo all over, then lathering, taking care to clean anal area, groin, under forelegs inside the pads on the feet. Massage the body well with your finger tips as this will really clean the skin and stimulate the circulation. Check the skin while the coat is wet, as it is easier to see signs of skin trouble then. Rinse off well, remembering to spray under the collar, and underneath the dog's body. Towel dry him very thoroughly and let him race around the garden to finish drying off. Obviously you should not bath your dog in cold weather, or even a cold summer day, in the garden.

Do not use ordinary human shampoo as this can cause a very bad reaction on your dog. Use a specially formulated dog shampoo such as Seleen, Sherley's Coatacine, Derasect to name but a few.

Do's and Dont's

1   Never ever leave chicken or poultry bones or indeed any cooked bones lying around, especially in the disposal bin in your kitchen. Dobermanns are dab hands at sussing out how to open bins and fridge doors. Put the bones firmly wrapped in your dustbin with the lid tightly sealed. Always make sure your garbage can in the kitchen is out of reach, you would be surprised what a hungry puppy will find to eat.

2   Another very important thing to watch in the kitchen is if, like us, you have a low grill on your cooker. It is just the right height for Dobermanns and manys the time I have had to rescue my husband's dinner which has been whipped from under the grill.

3   Never strike a puppy in anger and never punish him out of your own bad temper. Always be calm, temperate and deal with situations quickly and at the time they occur.

4   Do not throw sticks for puppy or even a grown dog to catch as if pounced on and caught in a certain way can cause great damage to your puppy/dog.

5   Do keep a nylon collar on the dog all the time, this makes it easy to hold the dog when visitors arrive.

6   Do keep the following household things out of an inquisitive puppy's way as they are all poisonous and very dangerous:
mothballs
aspirin, paracetamol and any other human drugs
bleach and dry cleaning fluid
laundry blue, nappy washes and soap powders
upholstery cleaners
antifreeze, brake fluids, petrol kerosene, motor oil
drain cleaners, garden sprays, insecticides
paint and paint thinners, (use lead free paint when decorating wherever possible)
weedkillers, slug bait and snail bait – NEVER USE

Care of an old Dobermann

Make life fun for your old dog, they ask very little from us, just adequate food, comfort, warmth and company.

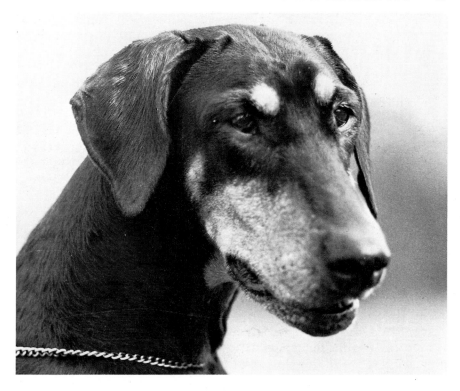

Ch Treasurequest
Cristal – an old
lady, full of dignity,
known as 'Helga',
2.11.70–21.11.84.
Owned by Stella
Law.

SIGHT

Sight degenerates with old age and also from a number of eye
diseases. If this happens try to keep things familiar for him in the
home. Do not move furniture around too much and keep him on
a lead when you take him for a walk.

HEARING

Some dogs go deaf with age but by this time your companion will
need few commands because he will have adjusted to doing what
you want by habit. You must of course take extra care of blind/
deaf dogs on the roads and clifftop walks and in other hazardous
situations.

INCONTINENCE

This becomes a problem with the older dog who may find it impossible to go through a ten hour night. It is only in very old age
that a dog will pass urine in its sleep. You may find you will have
to set up a routine similar to that of puppy days, either taking your

pet into your bedroom so it can wake you when it wants to go out, or cover the place he sleeps with newspaper which he can use.

Before you accept night frequency is due to old age, do ask your vet's advice since many dogs suffer with cystitis and kidney problems which clear up quickly after treatment. Be ready to adjust to your old friend's needs and never ever blame them if they are not as clean as they used to be as they cannot help it.

TEETH

Very aged dogs may appreciate their food being put through a liquidiser. Tinned food is excellent this way. An old dog can almost have a new lease of life by having troublesome teeth removed and some attention paid to the gums.

ODOUR

Reduced muscle tone in the intestine together with less inclination for exercise makes an old dog more prone to digestive trouble and to flatulence, noises and odours which can prove embarrassing to your company. Dobermanns have a way of walking away from a smell giving the owners reproachful glances as if to accuse them of making the awful smell themselves. A change of diet can sometimes help this problem.

ARTHRITIS

You may notice your old dog grunt with pain as he gets up and limps and staggers for the first few steps – this is the time to seek your vet's help.

This is common in old dogs and there is much help a vet can give to alleviate the pain and discomfort. Make sure his bed is especially soft as you will notice your Dobermann getting callouses on his elbows and hocks which can become very sore, if the surface that he lies on is too hard. Beanbags make excellent beds for arthritic dogs, providing them with warmth and support for their aching joints. The dog must not be rushed about, have lots of patience with him as he tries to hurry to you as quickly as he can.

HEART DISEASE

This is usually shown by a chronic cough and an inability to take much exercise. Be wary of the dog who is no longer keen to run and sits down while he is out. Your vet will advise you on medication and treatment to help your old friend.

POOR CIRCULATION

An ageing circulatory system can make an old dog feel the cold and if he cannot move fast enough to keep warm, put a warm coat on him for his last walk at night and also during very cold weather during the day.

OBESITY

Some dogs tend to get fat and excessive weight brings many problems, breathing difficulties, liver and skin problems and intolerance of hot weather. Prevention is better than cure so watch your dog's food intake in relation to its activity throughout its life.

MANAGEMENT

The cleverness and cunning of old dogs is something to be savoured and enjoyed to the fullest and it is a very special attribute in later life. Old age is most definitely a time for indulgence and spoiling, perhaps even letting them rule you a little.

FEEDING

After eight years of age reduce the red meat intake and replace it with fish, poultry and rabbit, adding a good wholemeal biscuit. Increase the biscuit until you are feeding biscuit only for several days of the week. Add parsley to the diet and barley water. Tinned tomatoes are especially good and a tablespoon a day will be sufficient. Oldies being less active need less food, but do split the meal into two meals a day.

EUTHANASIA

As everyone knows, time catches up with everyone and everything including our beloved pets. When the time comes and you realise that your old friend has reached the time in his life when he needs to go to his meadows in the skies, telephone your vet and arrange either for him to come to the house or for you to take your pet to him so that he can give him an injection which will put him to sleep, he will feel no pain and his last memory will be of you cuddling him. There are now many pet cemeteries and pet crematoria all over the country and if you have a word with your vet he will arrange for you to have your pet cremated and if you then want the ashes these are returned to you, to bury in your garden or sprinkle wherever his favourite place was. *Our Dogs* magazine holds a list of all the details of the cemeteries and crematoria in the country, so when you need this service write to them at the address below, send a stamped addressed envelope and you will be sent a list.

Our Dogs Publishing Company,
Oxford Road,
Station Approach
Manchester M60 1SX
Telephone 061 236 2660

6 The Bitch and Breeding

Seasons

When your bitch is coming into season, which normally happens twice a year at six monthly intervals she will need special care not to let her roam, or other dogs visit in your garden. You will notice that she puffs up behind and gradually swells up, starting to lose a dark blood discharge which is increased for a few days, and then gradually the colour changes to pink about the time the bitch is ready to ovulate. This is the time to take special care of your bitch as this is when she will feel the need to be mated, so be especially careful not to let her get out of the garden and equally important make certain that no dog can get into your garden. When you exercise her keep her on a lead – it won't hurt her not to have a free run for a couple of weeks. If you live in a very built up area do not take her out of your garden at all during that middle week as you will find all the dogs in the neighbourhood will be visiting.

The season usually lasts for about three weeks and it is in the middle week of this time that you have to be so careful. Seasons do vary however, and it is only by watching your bitch and perhaps noting down the time and as discharge changes colour that you will get some idea of the pattern of events. Seasons can also be quite messy. I usually put PETNIX or some other brand name of a type of panty on my bitches during this time but most bitches are very clean and look after themselves very hygenically. Another tip and one I always use is a product called NO STAIN. Use this if there are marks on the carpet. There are other products on the market but this is the one I have always used and am very satisfied with.

Should an accident occur, take your bitch to the vet within twenty-four hours for an injection.

One further piece of advice. Make a note of the date your bitch's season starts and then a further note six months further on, so you will have a rough idea of when she is next due and it won't come as such a surprise when she is in season again.

Phantom pregnancy

After a bitch has had her season, Dobermann bitches for some unknown reason tend to have a phantom pregnancy. Some phantoms are much worse than others and these obviously happen when a bitch has had her season and not been mated, or had a season, been mated and not had any puppies. It really is quite sad to see the bitch as she shows all the signs of pregnancy, some even have milk and they all go very maternal.

It is a question of seeing the bitch through this as gently as possible, giving her lots to do, so that she does not dwell on her thoughts, give her lots of exercise, don't leave her for long periods on her own, cut down a little on her food, don't give her any milk and cut down a little on her water. Give her plenty of toys to play with and keep her mind well occupied and she will probably not have such a bad phantom. However, some bitches do really have a bad time and if this becomes the case with your bitch then it is very wise to discuss treatment with your vet.

Breeding from your bitch

It is very important that you do not breed from your bitch before she is two years old. If you decide that you really do want to have a litter of puppies the best advice I can give you is to discuss this with the breeder of your bitch.

Do not use a dog just because he lives down the road and it is convenient. There is such an awful lot to take into consideration when breeding from your bitch and I strongly recommend that you leave this to the more experienced breeders until you know a good deal about the breed, about your bitch and her temperament and more importantly that the market for puppies is thoroughly investigated. I know from experience how many puppies are left unsold at about sixteen to twenty weeks, sometimes even longer than that. For the experienced breeder this may not be the end of the world as they usually have the facilities for keeping puppies and older dogs but for the novice breeder it can be an expensive disaster. For the puppies concerned it could be devastating and a very bad start to their lives, so please, until you have a good sound knowledge of the breed leave this part to the experienced breeder and enjoy your bitch for what she is and what you bought her for, a pet, companion and friend. I know a lot of people are told by their vet that it is best for the bitch to have just one litter but please believe me, this really is not the case.

There is nothing more worrying or soul destroying than trying to meet vet bills and food bills and staying in and looking after the bitch and her babies when you really want to go out, so please, think long and hard before making the decision to mate her.

When I first decided to write this book I did not want to write a full chapter on breeding as the breeding programme is so involved. This chapter only touches upon it lightly and not in any depth. It is hoped to give readers an insight into what breeding is all about but at the same time I would hope that they will follow my earlier advice and only breed when they have owned a Dobermann for some time.

I am grateful to the Findjans Kennels for their help, advice and guidance in putting this chapter together.

Most dogs are sexually mature and capable of mating a bitch by the time they are ten months old. It is most important that the dog has two normal descended testes and his other external genitalia are anatomically correct before contemplating using a dog at stud.

Whilst it may seem an attractive idea to mate your bitch with your friend's dog, you could be running into a lot of trouble because unless your friend is knowledgeable, the dog may not be, and management of a stud dog is most important. It is far better to take your bitch to a professional stud dog as he will be trained in this type of work. You should be able to see some of his offspring as well, which is so important. The stud dog owner could also mete out advice during your bitch's pregnancy about care of the young puppies.

It is best to seek the advice of the breeder of your bitch who will be pleased to suggest suitable dogs compatible to the pedigree of your bitch. Try also to choose a stud dog which is HD and CVI clear. The search for your stud dog should start early and you may change your mind about a dog several times before actually deciding but this can only be a good thing as it will show you are learning about type.

Before contemplating breeding find out all you can about your bitch's pedigree. Whelping ability is strongly hereditary and to attempt to breed from a bitch which has a history of problems (perhaps she was born by caesarian or was an only puppy whose mother refused to feed her) could be very unwise. If you bought your bitch as a pet and she was not technically a very good specimen as regards the standard it is not a good idea to breed from her, as some of her pups will carry on any faults and the breed then starts to degenerate. It is best to check with the breeder as to the suitability of breeding from her at the time of purchase. Some bitches which are sold as pets because they have known faults may be registered at the Kennel Club but could well be on the Non-Active Register and puppies from them wouldn't be eligible for registration.

If you do decide to breed it is best to talk to your vet and to start to get the bitch into the best possible condition for having a litter. Dobermanns should not be bred from until they are two years old and only then if they are calm and mature and never before the third season at the very earliest.

A bitch should always be tested for any infection before mating. During the first part of the season the bitch sometimes is high spirited or irritable. The vulva enlarges and softens and you will see a blood stained discharge. She will be ready for mating anytime between ten and fourteen days, but individual bitches vary greatly.

The most common reason for a bitch missing is that she is taken to be mated too early. Unless she is ready mentally and physically she will refuse to be mated. It is very wrong and cruel to force a mating with a bitch that is not ready. An experienced stud dog will only mate a bitch when he knows she is ready by her scent, even if she does present herself to him.

Stud procedure

It is usual for the bitch to visit the dog. Sometimes arrangements can be made to meet halfway and sometimes if the stud dog is confident he can be taken to the bitch, but the most usual way is for the bitch to go to the dog. A mating can be rather a tense business for the owner of the bitch as well as for the bitch.

Bitches are known to have preferences to a dog of their own choice. The stud fee should be paid at the time of mating and should be paid regardless whether puppies are born or not. You are paying for the service of the stud dog, although if a bitch misses most stud dog owners offer a return mating but this is not obligatory.

Some stud dog owners will allow two matings on alternate days, others allow only one. Most stud dog owners are professional and anxious for their reputation and that of their dog to be maintained. Some stud dog owners will take a puppy for a stud fee, this is usually done by a written agreement in exchange for the stud fee which is payable immediately a satisfactory mating has been obtained, the bitch's owner should be given a copy of the stud dog's pedigree with the Kennel Club number on and a form to register the litter. It is also important to receive a copy of an *HD* and *CVI* certificates, check that these certificates show the Kennel Club number of dog used. Keep a signed copy of any agreement made for a return stud, in case the bitch should miss.

The mating

Once you have decided to mate your bitch it is imperative that you get her into top condition. Check with the Kennel Club that her registration is valid so that the puppies will be eligible for registration. The bitch should be checked over by the vet for any skin diseases and she should have a swab taken and a course of antibiotics to clear any infection. She should also be receiving any vaccination boosters that will fall within the next four months which will enable her to pass on the maximum amount of antibody to her pups. The bitch should be wormed before mating. Make certain the bitch is on a feeding routine she accepts and start giving her a well balanced multi vitamin mineral preparation made by a reputable company. It is better to do this than to juggle and guess with cod liver oil, bonemeal etc which you have to be so careful and accurate in giving. Some breeders give Vitamin E as an aid to fertility but this should be started well before the expected day of mating. Watch your bitch for signs of coming into season. The first day she starts losing a blood-stained discharge is the time to start counting the days. Test her vulva with a kleenex each day as bitches do keep themselves very clean and could quite easily mislead you if you are not watching closely enough.

A minority of bitches have a colourless season which is an abnormality and although they can be mated and perhaps be fertile you would have to judge the day of mating by size and expansion of the vulva and the amount of sexual excitement the bitch is exhibiting.

On the first day the bitch shows colour you should phone the stud dog owner and make arrangements to take her. While waiting for the correct day to come round you must maje sure your bitch cannot get out of your garden or more importantly that strays cannot get in.

When you take your bitch to be mated do all you can to keep her from getting upset and do not feed her before taking her. Allow the bitch to empty her bladder before arriving at the stud dog's home and leave her in the car while you find the stud dog owner who will let you know where to take your bitch for the mating.

Bring your bitch in on a strong leather collar. The stud dog owner usually organises the mating. It is preferable to allow the dogs to free play and you will notice when the bitch is ready as she will stand with her tail to one side and her vulva uptilted. The bitch should be held and it may be necessary to muzzle her and it may also be necessary to have someone hold the bitch under the abdomen.

The dog ejaculates in three stages. The first is watery and contains no sperms and often has a characteristic odour. Then comes the sperm-bearing fraction but this should not be clear and thirdly a copious amount to wash the sperm upwards in the cervix of the bitch.

The ejaculatory part of the mating will be over in two to three minutes. Then comes the tie. As the bitch would be unable to bear the weight of the dog on her back he turns himself or is turned by the handlers so that the pair are back to back. A tie is obviously preferable but matings can be fertile without a tie provided dog and bitch have been in contact long enough for the sperm to be introduced. During the tie some bitches may cry, it is an emotional reaction, some twist and try to free themselves and they must be steadied. When the tie is finally broken both dog and bitch will lick and clean themselves. Both should then be rested. Preferably put your bitch back into the car which is familiar to her and do remember that when you get her home she will still be in season so she must be kept away from other dogs.

After a bitch has been mated and for the remainder of the season she will most likely lose a little discharge which is nothing to worry about unless it becomes excessive.

Pregnancy

For the first five weeks of pregnancy there should be no extra food given or any change made to the bitch's normal routine. You should however be taking extra care of your bitch in more subtle ways and making certain she does not pick up any infection. Avoid taking her to dog shows and exercise should be continued as normal.

Your vet should be able to tell you if she is pregnant between twenty-one and twenty-eight days but no later can these little lumps be felt. A bitch will often let you know she is pregnant by becoming more tranquil and affectionate but others stay the same.

You will notice after five weeks changes in the bitch. Her teats will become more prominent and pink and her body thickens. One very reliable sign is the vulva which stays soft and relaxed and has a sticky discharge. She may go off her food and be choosy what she eats. An average bitch will need about one third more than normal with vitamins and minerals in proportion. In the sixth and seventh weeks ten per cent added protein should be given and during the last two weeks twenty-five per cent added protein. The bitch's ration should be divided into several small meals. The enlarged uterus exerts pressure on the stomach and she is unable to hold the quantity of food needed. Give hard boiled egg yolks in modest quantities. Any illness should be reported to your vet. Exercise should be kept up except in very hot weather, rough play must be discouraged and the bitch should not be allowed to run up and down stairs.

Every bitch whether mated or not undergoes hormone changes after her season and Dobermann bitches for some unknown reason always seem to have phantom pregnancies. It is not always easy to distinguish in the early stages between phantom and real pregnancies. The most reliable sign of pregnancy is the movement of the whelps during the last week or ten days of pregnancy. Around the seventh week the heavily in whelp bitch will show a definite change in outline – this happens literally overnight when the folding of the uterine horns occur. When this takes place it is best to feed the bitch in small amounts several times a day as it will be difficult for her during the night having a full bladder to remain clean. She should be allowed to take as much exercise as she likes.

It is normal for a clear discharge to be present as whelping day draws near but any blood stained or green stained discharge you need to see a vet immediately.

At the five to six week stage when you are fairly confident that puppies are on the way you should gather all the equipment together and prepare a room where your bitch will have her puppies. You will need to have a whelping box made for the bitch to have her puppies in and where she can rear them for the first few weeks. An infra-red lamp is essential plus lots of newspapers and big black dustbin bags to put all the soiled newspapers in. Other important equipment is listed below:

A clock to time the interval between births
Notepaper and pen and scales to weigh each puppy and write weight down
Specially formulated milk
Torch
Glucose solution
Lubricant jelly
Kitchen roll
Soft towels
Thermometer
Scissors
Vet Beds
Kennel club forms for registering puppies
Pedigree forms
Diet sheets typed and duplicated.

The whelping room should have a good light and be near a source of water. It should be a warm and quiet spot away from distracting noises, people and other dogs. Introduce the bitch to her quarters at least ten days before she is due so that she can become accustomed to her new surroundings.

Whelping

A few days before whelping you will find your bitch is fidgety, uncomfortable and restless. Find out what the vet's arrangements are for emergency calls and how to reach him day and night. You should also have organised who will be doing the puppies' dew claws and tails. Some vets will do this, some will not, so then you should make sure someone in the breed will do it for you. A bitch in whelp likes the company of someone she trusts but the less you interfere the better. As the day draws near to your bitch having her puppies you will notice her vulva enlarging and softening. The bitch may refuse her food and if you have kept a twice a day temperature chart you will find her temperature will fall about two degrees to around ninety-nine degrees as whelping time draws near.

The bitch may shiver and pant and this can go on for some time. This is normal, during this stage the cervix will dilate and start to open to allow the puppies through and at this stage the bitch may want to tear up paper or bedding which is a natural reaction reverting back to nature of digging a hole to have her whelps in. The contractions can cause the bitch some distress. The main thing to look for at this stage is a green stained discharge. If this happens before a puppy is born it is imperative you get the vet and help urgently. Green watery discharge after a puppy or more has been born is normal.

Each puppy is attached by its placenta, the blood filled tissue that will come out with the puppy or just after it has been born. At the first contraction the bitch may cry and look around to see what is happening. You should comfort her and tell her what a clever girl she is. Note the time of the contraction as this will be important to the vet if he has to take any action. You must be ready to help the bitch by breaking the bag with your finger nails but make sure the puppy is breathing, wipe the nose and clear the inside of the mouth to drain out the mucus and do all of this beside the bitch so she can see what you are doing. You should dry the puppy as quickly as possible, let the bitch lick her and put her on a teat to get the colostrum which contains the antibodies which immunise the pups for a few weeks. Sometimes the bitch may really rough house the puppy around the whelping box, rolling it over with her nose. Do not be alarmed, this is nature's way of stimulating the puppy's circulation but can be a very frightening sight for a novice breeder.

GESTATION TABLE SHOWING WHEN A BITCH IS DUE TO WHELP

Served Jan.	Whelps March	Served Feb.	Whelps April	Served March	Whelps May	Served April	Whelps June	Served May	Whelps July	Served June	Whelps Aug.	Served July	Whelps Sept.	Served Aug.	Whelps Oct.	Served Sept.	Whelps Nov.	Served Oct.	Whelps Dec.	Served Nov.	Whelps Jan.	Served Dec.	Whelps Feb.
1	5	1	5	1	3	1	3	1	3	1	3	1	2	1	3	1	3	1	3	1	3	1	2
2	6	2	6	2	4	2	4	2	4	2	4	2	3	2	4	2	4	2	4	2	4	2	3
3	7	3	7	3	5	3	5	3	5	3	5	3	4	3	5	3	5	3	5	3	5	3	4
4	8	4	8	4	6	4	6	4	6	4	6	4	5	4	6	4	6	4	6	4	6	4	5
5	9	5	9	5	7	5	7	5	7	5	7	5	6	5	7	5	7	5	7	5	7	5	6
6	10	6	10	6	8	6	8	6	8	6	8	6	7	6	8	6	8	6	8	6	8	6	7
7	11	7	11	7	9	7	9	7	9	7	9	7	8	7	9	7	9	7	9	7	9	7	8
8	12	8	12	8	10	8	10	8	10	8	10	8	9	8	10	8	10	8	10	8	10	8	9
9	13	9	13	9	11	9	11	9	11	9	11	9	10	9	11	9	11	9	11	9	11	9	10
10	14	10	14	10	12	10	12	10	12	10	12	10	11	10	12	10	12	10	12	10	12	10	11
11	15	11	15	11	13	11	13	11	13	11	13	11	12	11	13	11	13	11	13	11	13	11	12
12	16	12	16	12	14	12	14	12	14	12	14	12	13	12	14	12	14	12	14	12	14	12	13
13	17	13	17	13	15	13	15	13	15	13	15	13	14	13	15	13	15	13	15	13	15	13	14
14	18	14	18	14	16	14	16	14	16	14	16	14	15	14	16	14	16	14	16	14	16	14	15
15	19	15	19	15	17	15	17	15	17	15	17	15	16	15	17	15	17	15	17	15	17	15	16
16	20	16	20	16	18	16	18	16	18	16	18	16	17	16	18	16	18	16	18	16	18	16	17
17	21	17	21	17	19	17	19	17	19	17	19	17	18	17	19	17	19	17	19	17	19	17	18
18	22	18	22	18	20	18	20	18	20	18	20	18	19	18	20	18	20	18	20	18	20	18	19
19	23	19	23	19	21	19	21	19	21	19	21	19	20	19	21	19	21	19	21	19	21	19	20
20	24	20	24	20	22	20	22	20	22	20	22	20	21	20	22	20	22	20	22	20	22	20	21
21	25	21	25	21	23	21	23	21	23	21	23	21	22	21	23	21	23	21	23	21	23	21	22
22	26	22	26	22	24	22	24	22	24	22	24	22	23	22	24	22	24	22	24	22	24	22	23
23	27	23	27	23	25	23	25	23	25	23	25	23	24	23	25	23	25	23	25	23	25	23	24
24	28	24	28	24	26	24	26	24	26	24	26	24	25	24	26	24	26	24	26	24	26	24	25
25	29	25	29	25	27	25	27	25	27	25	27	25	26	25	27	25	27	25	27	25	27	25	26
26	30	26	30	26	28	26	28	26	28	26	28	26	27	26	28	26	28	26	28	26	28	26	27
27	31	27	1	27	29	27	29	27	29	27	29	27	28	27	29	27	29	27	29	27	29	27	28
28	1	28	2	28	30	28	30	28	30	28	30	28	29	28	30	28	30	28	30	28	30	28	1
29	2	29	3	29	31	29	1	29	31	29	31	29	30	29	31	29	1	29	31	29	31	29	2
30	3			30	1	30	2	30	1	30	1	30	1	30	1	30	2	30	1	30	1	30	3
31	4			31	2			31	2			31	2	31	2			31	2			31	4

Normally a bitch will carry her puppies from sixty-two to sixty-three days but even if she goes three days more or less than this time there is no cause for alarm. The table set out above should therefore be taken as a general guide and not as a rigidly fixed timetable.

Allow the bitch to eat only two or three placenta and take the rest away as too many will give her diarrhoea. The bitch should never be allowed to go longer than two hours and produce nothing. During the course of the time the bitch is whelping she will appreciate an occasional drink of milk and water with a little glucose and this is best given in between her having the pups. You must also watch for inertia and in some lines this is more likely to occur if there has been a history of this. If your vet asks you to bring her into the surgery do not panic, wrap her in a blanket, if there is inertia the drive will encourage the bitch to start pushing again. When the whelping has finished your first job will be to take the bitch outside while someone else removes all the soiled newspaper and puts in fresh, clean vet beds or newspapers.

Immediately after whelping give a raw egg beaten in milk and glucose and later on feed her a good quality light diet of chicken. Offer this to her in the whelping box as she will be reluctant to leave her new babies. She should be fed little and often, feed her according to her demand, most nursing bitches are ready for their usual meat and biscuits but she should drink plenty of milk and/or water and her diet should now include extra meat, eggs, vitamins and calcium.

The bitch will have a discharge which may go on for a few weeks. Any tarry black offensive discharge needs immediate veterinary attention. It is wise to have the vet in soon after whelping to give her an injection to make sure all the placenta and mess inside her has come out. This injection can wait until the morning. You should already have made arrangements for tails and dew claws to be done and this is best carried out when the bitch is out of the room as the puppies crying will upset her.

You must watch your bitch very carefully for eclampsia which is caused by an imbalance of calcium that is essential to life and can still occur even though you have been feeding calcium regularly. The signs vary but the bitch's reaction is quite bizarre. The bitch must never be left long unattended after having a litter. If you suspect eclampsia (see glossary) you must get the vet whatever time of day or night it is.

Another problem that could occur is mastitis. The first signs will be a swelling and hard lumps in the mammary glands. This is caused by a bug that causes infection. Veterinary advice is a must as the bitch could lose all her milk and a painful ulcer could break open.

It is a good idea to weigh the puppies at birth and every week thereafter to make sure they are holding their own and inspect them initially to see if there are any abnormalities present, cleft palate, mal formed joints etc.

The puppies' eyes should open at about ten days. All eyes are blue at first and change as the puppies grow. From ten days onwards the bitch will be eating all she can and it will be virtually impossible to over feed her. She will need three to four times more than her usual feed with vitamins and minerals in proportion. Do not use fly sprays around puppies, use the good old fashioned sticky fly paper.

When the puppies are three weeks old they will be struggling to get on their feet and their hearing then is very sharp. They can also bark. At about three weeks of age the puppies should be walking about. Their eyes should be open and they should be able to hear. From twenty-one days onwards puppies must socialise and be seen and handled by people and become familiar with household noises, bangs and crashes, radio, television, and vacuum cleaners. The puppies should be in a busy room with lots of traffic passing through and a run and shelter in the garden for during the day. The more room they have the cleaner they will become, but a puppy run is essential. Puppies need to sleep a lot and be allowed to have all the rest they need so do ensure that there are regular periods when they are not disturbed.

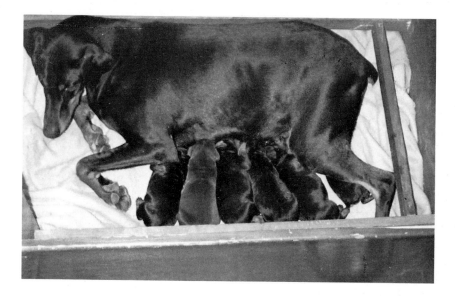

The Milk Bar.

Once you have started feeding the puppies on meat the bitch will stop cleaning up after them. It is also very interesting to see how the bitch teaches her puppies from walking and running to looking after themselves in a dangerous situation. This early learning is important to a puppy as if he is sold as a solitary pet he will probably have no other opportunity to learn to defend himself. The bitch's behaviour with her pups teaches us a lot. If they pull her ears or persist in annoying her when she wants to sleep she will snap once decisively and her puppies, impressed by her behaviour, stop what they are doing to annoy her, in surprise. All puppy training should be modelled on this.

Weaning puppies begins as soon as their teeth are through at about four weeks of age. Pedigree Chum Puppy Food is an ideal start to your puppies diet as it is completely balanced and nothing extra in the way of vitamins and minerals is required.

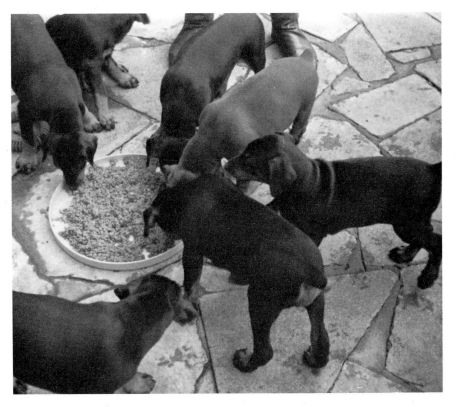

Meal times.

Feed all the puppies from one dish as competition seems to stimulate them. It can be very difficult with a very large litter to get a dish large enough, in this case feed with two dishes and put equal numbers of pups to each dish.

Puppies must be watched closely all the time. Disabilities do begin to show at the time of weaning. At five weeks all puppies must be able to stand, see, hear and run. By the time the puppies are seven to eight weeks they should be on four meals a day and they should have been wormed regularly.

Puppies must not be allowed to endure bowel weakness as it is very weakening and dehydrating so if the condition persists for more than twenty-four hours get your vet's advice.

As the puppies' food is increased so the bitch's food should be decreased and her exercise increased. She should be wormed again. The puppies' nails should be clipped every week while they are in the nest.

A rough guide to an average weight of dog and bitch puppies is as follows:

At one week bitches weigh 1lb 6oz (.6kg) and the dogs 1lb 5oz (.59kg)

At two weeks the bitches weigh 2lb 9oz (1.16kg) and the dogs 2lb 7oz (1.11kg)

At three weeks the bitches weigh 3lb 6oz (1.53kg) and the dogs 3lb 4oz (1.47kg)

At four weeks the bitches weigh 4lb 12oz (2.15kg) and the dogs 4lb 8oz (2.04kg)

At six weeks dogs take over and are about 2oz (57g) heavier than the bitches, with dogs weighing about 8lb 4oz (3.74kg) and bitches 8lb 2oz (3.68kg)

At eight weeks of age the difference is often as much as 8oz (456g) the dogs weighing about 12½lb (5.7kg) and the bitches around 12lb (5.4kg).

At one year Dobermanns are nearly fully grown, but then start filling out and maturing, although some dogs take quite a time to mature whilst others are mature as puppies. Some bitches at that age are really grown up and mature, whilst others of the same age still look like babies and very immature. The dogs and bitches put on weight in bone, although not necessarily becoming fatter.

Selling your puppies

The stud dog owner may be able to pass on enquiries to you but the Dog Breeders' Association attracts the serious buyers.

It is important to let people visit several times and this makes things as certain as you can be that they are not impulse buyers. When you have finally checked out their suitability they should be requested to keep the puppy on the same diet, be given a certificate of worming and advice on how to proceed in the future.

Ask the new owners to take the puppy to the vet for a health check at the time of purchase. This covers the new owners and the breeder on the puppy's health. It is also the best way to start up a contact with the vet who will also advise on a vaccination programme and be looking after the dog, probably for the rest of his life. A parvo virus injection is normally given at six weeks of age but you should check with your vet for his thoughts on this.

If you choose to charge the same prices as the top breeders for your puppies then you must be prepared to give a top service care and after care to help the new owners. Raising and rearing a litter of Dobermann puppies is expensive and very hard work, worthwhile and rewarding at the best, but soul destroying, devastating and depressing if things go wrong. Breeders have a grave responsibility to the little lives they create.

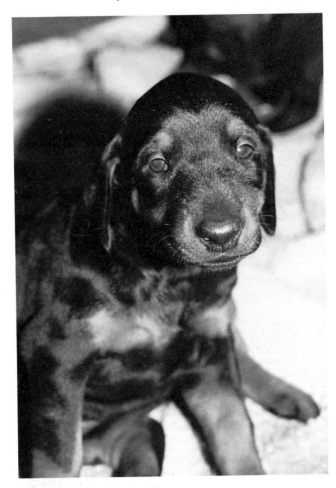

Puppy head – a trusting 3 week old puppy.

One other thing, never sell your puppies overseas to the Far East and countries that do not show or know the value of this lovely breed. They deserve more than a life of pain and suffering and starvation that could be their doom if they are sent abroad to certain countries.

7 Training

Basic principles

Colonel Konrad Most, writing in *Training Dogs*, describes the way to a mutual understanding between man and dog and I am grateful to him and his publishers for their permission to quote from his book: 'From childhood onwards we are taught a great deal that is wrong about the psychology of animals. In fables, fairy tales and stories describing animal life and behaviour we are often presented with living beings that think, understand human speech and perform moral or immoral acts. If we adopt these anthropomorphic views we shall be at a disadvantage whenever we try to train animals of any kind, but particularly when we are dealing with dogs.

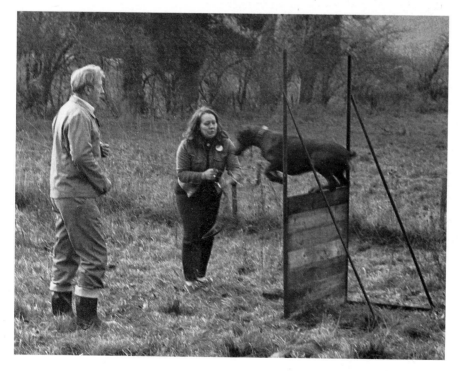

Learning to jump the scale.

'We can save ourselves much disappointment and ensure the dog's more rapid and cheerful response to instruction by allowing him to learn in the canine way.

'The dog most closely resembles man in his emotional and instinctive reflexes. He is capable of showing his emotions very eloquently and his manner of expressing his feelings is clearly reflected in our own.

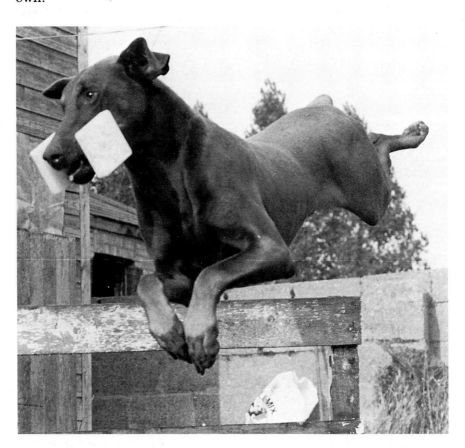

Working Dobermanns: Vyleighs Mustang who is also a TV and Film Star. Owned by Heidi Vyse.

'It is responses of this kind that largely account for our deep affection for dogs. We are so impressed by the acuteness of such senses as those of scent and hearing, and with the capacity to learn, that we are prone to assume that a dog's mental equipment approximates to our own. We credit him with capacity for thought and with an understanding of human behaviour and morality. By introducing the dog into a world which is, in reality, for ever closed to him, we prevent ourselves from recognising the unbridgeable mental gap that exists between man and dog.'

Training to come when called

All training is a matter of repetition and always using the same command words. Whilst playing with your puppy watch him running about and he will most probably run away from you and then turn and run back to you. Say 'come' in an encouraging voice. Never use a demanding or scolding tone for this. When he comes, tell him how clever he is, pat him and make a fuss. Occasionally when called give him a titbit and he will soon learn that it is pleasant to come to you. Keep this training up until he is really good at coming to you and it will soon become a habit to come to your call.

However, not all things go as smoothly as we would like and if your dog is difficult to recall, you may find yourself standing around for ages (usually in the pouring rain) while he toddles off to do his own thing and just won't come back. This is the time when you have to grit your teeth and summon up all the self restraint you can muster, so that you can greet him with a pat and a 'good dog' when he does eventually return.

Never be angry or smack him, no matter how long you have to wait. If the problem still continues, make sure that when he is running free and he comes up to greet you, you pat him and then send him away again to play. Never let him think he is going to be trapped. With a Dobermann surprise is the element, NEVER let him know what you are thinking.

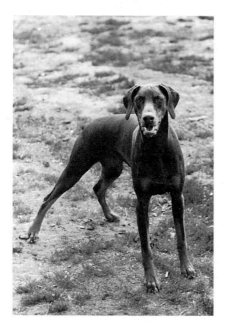

W T Ch Linrio Domingo CDx, UDx, WDx, TDx, PDx, Winner of the Kennel Club Championship Tracking Stake. Despite setbacks as a youngster and losing 9 months from the trials circuit, after only her second year in trials and winning her first ticket, Rio achieved Top Working Dobermann, and is the highest qualified Dobermann ever in the UK. She has won ASPADS Tracker Dog of the Year in 1983 and 1985 plus the Kennel Club Championship Working Trial (Tracking Stake) for 1984/85. Bred by Mr & Mrs Arnott. Owned and trained by Mr J. Middleweek.

Training to walk to heel

When your puppy has learned to wear a collar and lead begin to teach him to walk to heel. Start off with the puppy on your left side, the end of the lead in your right hand. The left hand goes on the lead only when you jerk the dog to you.

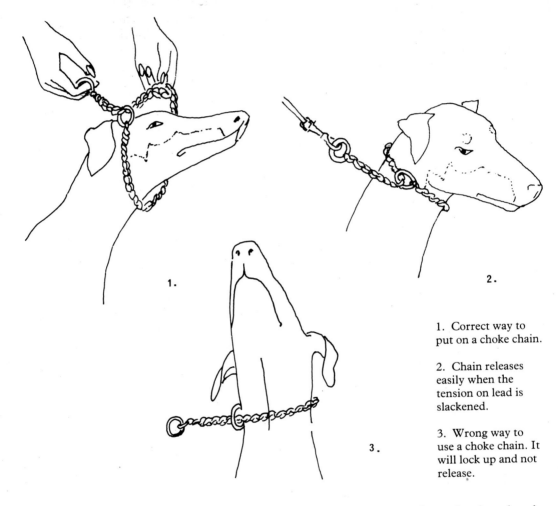

1.

2.

3.

1. Correct way to put on a choke chain.

2. Chain releases easily when the tension on lead is slackened.

3. Wrong way to use a choke chain. It will lock up and not release.

The art of getting a dog to heel is to have a loose lead and only check him when he pulls away from you. He may drag behind, or once having gained his confidence, he will most likely pull ahead. A dragging puppy must be encouraged with kind words until he will keep up. The one who pulls ahead has to learn that he must stay at his owner's side.

Puppies should be treated gently and given plenty of encouragement. The use of the lead to correct the pup as in fig 2 should always coincide with the command 'heel'.

An upward jerk with both hands on the lead accompanied by the command 'heel' will pull the puppy to your side. Walk fairly smoothly in a square and when you turn right or left always bring the dog to heel after you have turned. Repeat as necessary and they soon get the idea of what is required. A ten minute session of right and left turns a day should give the puppy the idea of the exercise. Immediately your puppy obeys caress his/her head. Praise is a most important part of training the Dobermann.

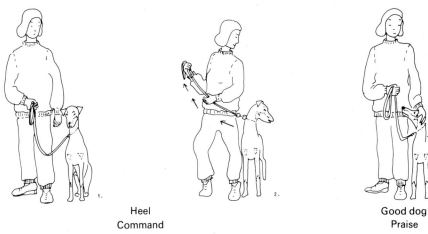

Heel
Command

Good dog
Praise

Training to sit

These diagrams show the correct way to teach the dog to sit when it is told.

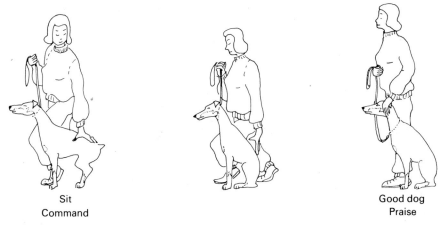

Sit
Command

Good dog
Praise

Car travelling

Some puppies are car sick, others dribble and drool alarmingly, usually this is caused by nerves, but in any case it is advisable to sit puppy on an old rug or some newspapers to protect the seat. Take him for short distances only to start with. After a few days he should get over his sickness and begin to look forward to his car rides, especially when he associates a ride in the car with something special at the end, like a run in the park or woods.

Give him something to chew to take his mind off the car and never take him out in the car just after feeding him. If the sickness is very bad give the puppy 'Sealegs' or 'Vetzyme' 'Easy Travel' These are known and effective treatments.

When the puppy is used to the car it may not be necessary to continue with Sealegs or Easy Travel – don't despair the problem will right itself – eventually.

Leaving a puppy alone

There should be some period or periods during the day when your puppy is left on its own. If he always has human company with him he will expect this all the time and may grow to dislike being left on his own so that when you go out and cannot take him you will need a dog sitter, much as children have to have a baby sitter.

If you start when he is a very young puppy and leave him to sleep after he has eaten and done his business in the garden, then it should come quite naturally for him to be left as he will be used to being put away for a little nap. Always leave him with plenty of toys and his water bowl. You will find you can extend the time he is left as he gets older and more confident and he will know the routine.

Ringcraft and obedience classes

Keeping in mind that this book is primarily for the new or prospective Dobermann owner, the full meaning of 'working dog' may not be immediately apparent to the reader. After a few weeks of attending training classes, many new owners become 'hooked' on training and working their new pals and even begin to set their sights on competing in the obedience ring or going on to working trials, hoping to gain one or more of the following titles to add to their dog's name:

C.D.	Companion Dog	U.D.	Utility Dog
W.D.	Working Dog	T.D.	Tracker Dog

To which, with a lot of hard work and patience, maybe added 'X' (for excellent) to those titles listed.

Even if these objects are, for some reason or other, never achieved, the challenge of working a truly independent and intelligent animal is a pleasure in itself. The new friends found amongst others who also strive to get the best from themselves and their super-dog partners, are an extra perk. As handlers we have to learn to understand the dog's natural ability to do all we ask of it, but also to realise that we may not always ask in a way the dog understands.

Because of the sheer power and strength of this breed training is of the utmost importance, but training by the right type of trainers.

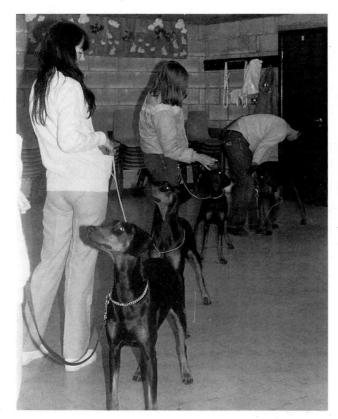

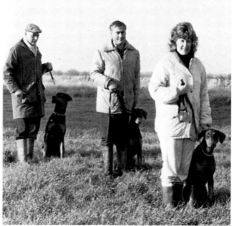

Obedience training classes.

Ringcraft training classes.

Most Dobermanns can be trained adequately at obedience classes and in some areas there are special classes for Dobermanns only. It is most unwise to send your dog away for training as you need to be trained together. It is of no use whatsoever to send your Dobermann away because when he comes back to you you will both need to work together and learn together for the training to be effective, and this obviously will not happen if you send him away on his own – besides which, you want to know exactly how your Dobermann is being treated. Advice on training should always be sought from experienced, knowledgeable people who are well respected in the breed.

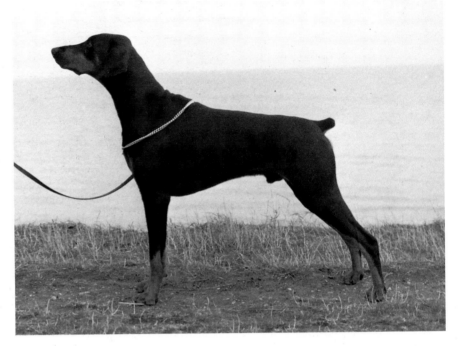

Ch Perihelias Resolution. Owned by Mr & Mrs Bartle.

8 Showing

The novice and showing

It may be a chance remark from a stranger who admires your beautiful Dobermann that starts you thinking how much you would love to show him off and let others see what a lovely dog you have. Or perhaps as you are walking in the country watching your fabulous Dobermann running back and forth, breathtakingly beautiful, chasing through the trees, running far and wide and dashing up to tell you something he has seen, his fine enquiring face alive with beauty and character you say to yourself 'I must show him'.

You may be lucky to know somebody who shows their dogs who can advise you. If you don't, then start by buying *Dog World* or *Our Dogs* (these are the two dog papers and usually have to be ordered through your newsagent) and look up the shows in your area.

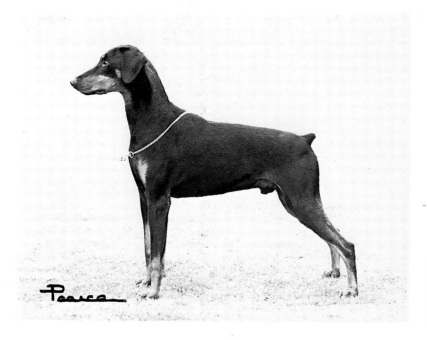

Ch Javictreva Brief Defiance of Chater. Bred by N. Simmons. Owned by Mrs V. Philip

Send for a schedule and then complete the entry form. Your dog must be registered at the Kennel Club in order for you to show at any Kennel Club event and over six months of age. Some shows are held on one, two or even three days and you must be sure if it is more than a one day show that you attend on the correct day as Dobermanns are included in the Working Group. There are six groups: working, hounds, terriers, utility, toys and gundogs.

Exemption shows are a very good start for the novice and a lot of fun and a good day out for the whole family, as well as being very good practice for your puppy and you before embarking on the trials and tribulations of a show of a more competitive nature. You may see variety classes advertised in the schedule. To enter these classes you must first be entered in the breed class, the variety class being for dogs of all breeds competing against one another.

If it is an open show there are usually only puppy novice graduate and open classes to enter. In some instances there are minor puppy and junior classes scheduled at an open show, but not all that often. At a championship show, there are usually minor puppy, puppy, novice, junior, post graduate limit and open, for each sex. Puppy classes are from six months to twelve months on the day of the show, and then you go into the next class up. Minor puppy ages are six to nine months, so be sure to enter the right class and do not make the mistake of entering the puppy in more than puppy and perhaps novice. When you have filled in the entry form send it off within the deadline for closing date.

Take your dog to ring craft classes where you will be taught how to handle properly and shown how to move the dog correctly and to its best advantage both in a triangle and in a straight line up and down. It is necessary to move your dog correctly to enable the judge to assess its movement. Practice everything you have been taught at these classes, socialise your puppy in every way you can and get him used to every possible situation.

You will need a fine choke chain 28″ to 30″ (710 to 760mm) long, (finer than the one you use every day) and a fine lead. Trim your dog's whiskers around his face and his eyebrows, trim his nails every week and use a thick rubber glove (bought from a pet shop) to remove dead hair daily. A velvet glove or a piece of velvet is ideal to keep with you in the ring just to add a final shine to his coat before the judge goes over him.

At an open show you can keep your dog with you, unless it is an extremely large open show when it will be, like all championship shows, benched. Benched means you have to put your dog on a bench partitioned off in sections approximately 2′6″ × 2′6″ (760mm × 760mm) on each side and your dog stays there all day except when you take him out to exercise him and to show him in the ring. At first you will need to stay with your puppy on the bench until he gets used to it after which he can safely be left on his own but it is always wise to keep an eye on him and not leave him for very long. You will need to put on the bench a blanket to sit on and secure him with a leather collar and a proper benching chain. He will also need a bowl of water and a favourite toy to keep him amused.

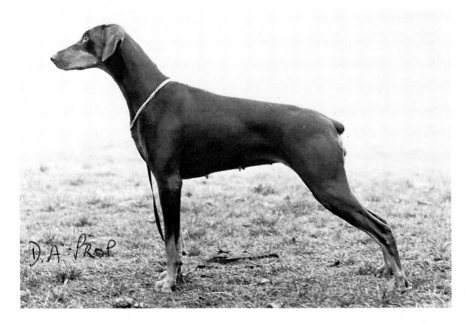

Ch Ashdobes Brown Berry. Bred and owned by Mrs S. Mitchell.

You enter the class applicable to the dog's age and sex. The routine in the ring is very similar to that of your ring craft classes. You enter the ring and the steward will give you a card with your number on, (at some shows this might be left on your bench). The steward will tell you where to stand and you stand your dog as you have been taught, keeping your eye on the judge and hopefully showing your dog to its best advantage while the judge walks round the ring for a first general assessment. The judge then sees each dog individually. When it is your turn you take your dog out in front of the judge and set him up, after the judge has gone over him, move him as requested, then join the line of other dogs until all exhibits have been seen. The steward usually lets you all know when the last dog is being seen and that is your cue to sort your dog out and get him looking his very best for the final assessment. If you are called out keep showing your dog right up until the placings are final – you could lose or gain places at the last moment.

Whether you win or lose always praise your puppy. As long as your puppy behaves and shows well and does his or her best you can ask no more of them. To win is a bonus and remember he is still the same puppy you brought out with you in the morning and is the same puppy you will be taking home and it is what they are like at home that is more important than winning.

Essentials for a show winter or summer are wet weather gear and wellingtons. In hot weather you will need comfortable clothes, water bowl and a towel, grooming kit, a chew for your dog on the bench and titbits (bait).

One important thing to remember if you have booked an open show and your bitch should be in season is that it is better not to go along as open shows are almost always mixed classes and it is not fair on the dogs in the class. A championship show is not so bad as usually there are separate rings for dogs and bitches.

With all shows it is important to adhere to the time the show starts. With championship shows in particular you must abide by the time of arrival and the departure time outlined in the schedule. This is a K.C. ruling and must be strictly adhered to.

9   The Owner's Responsibilities

The main responsibilities of any dog owner are to feed and groom your animal, to see a vet whenever necessary and take on the obligation of making your new dog part of your family for ever.

It is the owner's responsibility to let the dog know he is loved and wanted and to give him that feeling of safety and security he needs.

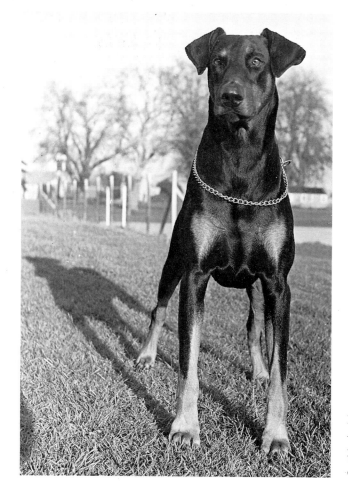

Barrimilne Black Adder. Bred by Mrs M. Bastable. Owned by Mr & Mrs Clements.

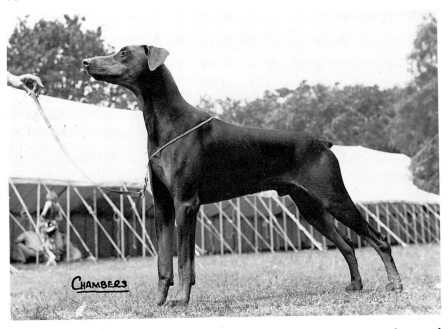

Dartrians Red
Arrow. Bred by Mrs
J. Storey. Owned by
Mrs J. Storey and
Mr K. Hood.

You should have at least third party insurance on your dog and
ensure that he has a collar and identity disc giving your address and
telephone number. If possible it is wise to have him tattooed. Do not
forget that you require a dog licence and you should have him vaccinated annually.

Do not allow your dog to harrass other people and their dogs
because this only adds to the myth of the 'vicious Dobermann'.
Always treat other people and their dogs with the utmost respect
and behaviour which is befitting that of the Dobermann, even if the
offenders are bad tempered and ill mannered.

Do not allow your dog to worry sheep or livestock. Apart from the
farmer being lawfully allowed to shoot any animal worrying his livestock, there is also the potential danger of the dog being kicked or
trampled on. Keep your dog under control at all times and on a lead
anywhere near a road or a farm.

Never allow your dog to foul public pavements or children's play
areas.

It is your responsibility to make sure that when travelling in a car
the dog is properly under control and never in a situation where he
can distract your driving. A new law has been passed about this and
there is a very hefty fine if caught.

Never try to bring in an animal from abroad or try to take your pet
abroad with you, without first seeing your vet regarding the very
strict laws on the Quarantine and Rabies Act 1974.

A dog's needs

It is not a good idea even to contemplate buying a Dobermann unless you have some garden or open space where he can run free and exercise himself. However dutiful you may be about taking the dog out a minimum of six times a day, in all weathers, it would impose too many restrictions on the dog. It would not be able to choose for itself when it wanted to be outside and never able to potter about looking for things that dogs look for and if you were ill and really couldn't get out what would happen?

Fencing must be of maximum height and gates secure and out of reach of children who could inadvertently open the gate and let the dogs run out and into the traffic.

Puppies and dogs do not do well if they are left for hours alone. They become bored, lonely, noisy and destructive. You cannot teach a puppy good behaviour unless you are there to correct it when it goes wrong or praise it when it does well. It is absolutely unacceptable for the breeder to let a puppy go to a home where someone works mornings only. This situation is unacceptable since human nature being what it is the dog will not be exercised and therefore tired enough before the family leaves for work in the morning. It takes a very strong-willed and dedicated person to exercise the dog early in the morning, perhaps not so bad in the summer when the mornings are light but in the winter months it will become a real bind. A four hour morning session at work often goes into six hours away from home by the time the shopping has been done.

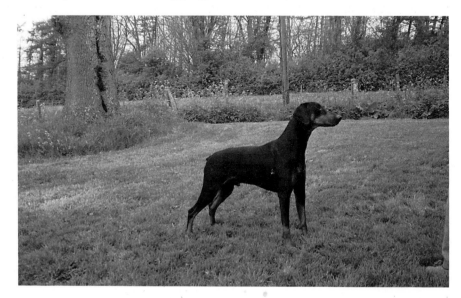

Chornytan Midnite Mark, 31.1.1976–28.5.1985. Sire of 4 Champions. Winner of the Royaltain 20th Anniversary Cup for Top Stud Dog 1981 and 1984. One of his sons, Chornytan Ace of Spades, is with Lincolnshire Police. *Daily Express* Pup of the Year Winner.

Never leave a dog in a stationary car in the summer as on a hot day the car heats up to a cruel 100°F + temperatures which can only be registered on a sugar thermometer. A car left in the shade at midday can be in full sunlight by 12.45 p.m. and your dog can become the victim of heat stroke and even death. Always therefore leave sufficient ventilation at any other time of the year for your dog. Remember the animals are in sheer panic trying to escape from what can only be described as a furnace.

Pets at holiday time

When you are making plans for your holiday you must also bear in mind at the same time what will happen to your pet whilst you are away. If you decide that you will all holiday together do make sure when you arrange your holiday that it is quite in order for you to take your pet along with you. There is a publication available from most newsagents called *Pets Welcome* which lists holiday accommodation where pets are accepted. Do make sure your pet wears his collar all the time and that the identity disc has the right address and telephone number – if you have recently moved house this is a very important job to remember to have done straight away.

Not all dogs travel well and it would be wise if it is a very long journey to seek your vet's advice on whether tranquillisers should be given. Always carry water for your pet and stop quite frequently to give him some exercise. Never let him off his lead. It is advisable to fix a proper dog guard in your car as windows can be left open without the dog jumping out. Never leave your dog in a car in hot weather.

On arrival at your holiday destination make sure you have the telephone number of the local vet, just in case of an emergency. Also remember that not everyone loves animals so please be sure they do not make or become a nuisance to anyone.

Should you decide that you prefer to board your pet in kennels, it is important to go and see the kennels first and decide that they are reliable and caring and a place you would like to leave your pet. It is best to seek advice and preferably recommendation of the kennels. Ask to see the accommodation offered and determine the charges and conditions of boarding. Make sure you meet the proprietor of the kennels personally as this will tell you a lot about the place. You will need up-to-date and full innoculation certificates and nowadays kennels are asking that dogs be innoculated against Kennel Cough. You will normally be required to pay a booking fee on reserving the accommodation which is not refundable but is credited to your account.

Accounts must be settled in full at the time you collect your pet. With some reputable kennels you are able to insure your pet whilst in their care.

There are several organisations which can provide you with advice on boarding kennels in your area:

Your local RSPCA
The local council
The National Boarding Kennels Association
C/o Blue Grass Animal Hotel,
Little Leigh,
Northwich,
Cheshire

National Canine Defence League
10 Seymour Street,
London W1H 5WB

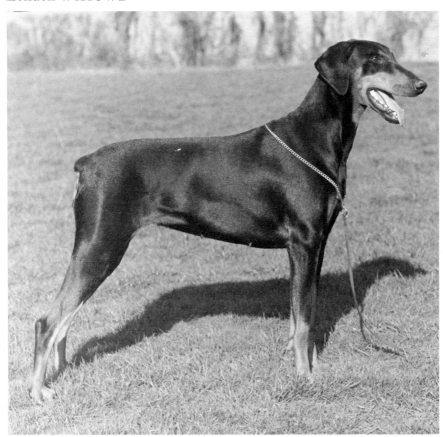

Ch Borains Raging Calm. Bred by Pat Gledhill. Winner of 17 C.C.s, 14 with Best of Breed. Bitch C.C. equal record holder. Twice Best of Breed at Crufts and only Dobermann Bitch to win a Reserve Group at Crufts.

Finally, should you decide to leave your pet with friends only do this if you are absolutely certain that the animal will be welcomed and properly looked after. Make sure your pet has an identity disc on with the address and telephone number of the person looking after him. Make sure your friend knows how to feed your dog, his little fads and that they also have the telephone number of your vet and of a local vet in the case of an emergency.

In the event of your illness or death

Although a subject one would obviously not want to think about it is important that in the case of sudden illness, accident or death your pet will be cared for immediately, without being caused any further distress than is necessary.

It takes only a few minutes to write down what should happen to your Dobermann, in fact any of your pets, and at least you will know you have done the very best for them. Provide definite instructions on feeding and keep a record of your dog's medical history, this eliminates the further suffering of the animal in your untimely death or illness. Put this information somewhere where it will be found easily or with a neighbour or friend.

Keep written records of your dog, these can prove invaluable if you have to use another vet away from your area in an emergency. Try and carry an RSPCA card with you at all times.

Dobermann Rescue

Dobermann Rescue was founded as an informal rescue organisation in 1967. It was registered in March 1984 as a company having no share capital but limited by guarantee. It is non-profit making and all its income is dedicated to its objectives, which are to organise the rescue and future welfare of Dobermanns in need; to give shelter to lost Dobermanns and to find good homes for them; to raise funds for these objectives.

There are many reasons for people not wanting to keep their dogs. There are always the genuine sad cases for having to put a precious Dobermann on Rescue, but there are many other thoughtless excuses, not least of all being 'the puppy has grown too big' it 'eats too much' and 'costs too much'. Dogs are not bought or sold by Rescue, but donations offered on putting dogs into care or on rehousing them and any offers of help with the cost of kennelling and running the organisation are gratefully received. The Rescue organisation is run by the council of the company and a band of dedicated helpers.

If for some reason you cannot keep your dog, don't give him away to anyone, don't be cruel to him because you don't want him any-more, give Dobermann Rescue a ring and they will try to rehouse your dog in the most suitable home. If you have just grown tired and fed up with your pet, please take this action. Rescue at least can rehome your once loved pet and you do at least owe him that much. Only ever deal with *bona fide* Rescue people, all of whom carry an identity card which you should always ask to see.

Perhaps you feel you could give a Rescue dog a good home; they may suit your circumstances better for whatever reason, and there are always dogs of varying ages needing a home. Yours may well be the one a Dobermann is looking for.

Some menus for dogs

BARLEY WATER

This is especially good for older dogs. Boil together pearl barley and water and then strain and give to dog once it has cooled.

BISCUITS

3lb (1·36kg) wholemeal plain flour
8oz (227g) dripping/fat
1 teaspoon cod liver oil
$\frac{1}{2}$ teaspoon salt
stock or beef cube
Mix to a stiff dough, roll out to $\frac{1}{2}$in (13mm) thick, cut into squares and bake in a medium oven for $\frac{1}{2}$ hour until golden brown.

CANINE COOKIES

2 small jars of beef baby food
2 small jars of chicken baby food
6oz (170g) wheatgerm and two eggs
Mix together and drop out on a cookie sheet. Bake at 350° for ten minutes. These can also be microwaved.

MISCELLANEOUS RECIPES

A chicken carcass or giblets cooked in stock water in a pressure cooker for at least an hour until the bones are very soft (removing any that are not) and put in a basin and left overnight to set will make a good jelly.

Brown wholemeal bread baked in the oven is a tasty change from regular meal and boiled brown rice unwashed is a good change from biscuits and very good for adding body.

Complan mixed with breakfast cereals is very good for dogs recovering from illnesses or general lack of appetite. Try the chocolate flavour.

Honey and glucose in warm milk is another good appetiser.
Cut stale wholemeal bread into thick half slices and crisp in a slow oven. These can be fed dry or broken and mixed with other food. They should be stored in airtight tins.

BONES

A Dobermann loves nothing better than a great big, juicy marrow bone. A good bone will last him ages. When it is temporarily abandoned rinse it in hot water, wipe it and dry it in a slow oven for a few minutes (don't cook it as it will make it brittle and dangerous). These big marrow bones help to keep your dog's teeth clean and strong. Never give any cooked bones, only marrow bones.

COLD WEATHER SPECIAL

Mix together one part liver, two parts melts and three parts cooked oatmeal porridge. This is a good complete meal in itself and you can add optional additives.

RECIPES FOR AN ELDERLY DOG

A Good Basic Feed
Mix together 4oz cooked cereal (oatmeal, wheat or brown rice) 4oz chopped or minced raw meat, 1 chopped hard boiled egg and a tablespoon of cottage cheese. Moisten with a little broth and serve at blood heat.

Beef pudding
Mince 1½lb lean beef scraps or ox heart and mix with 1½lb wholemeal flour and sufficient stock to make into a moist paste. Put in a basin and cover with a cloth. Steam for 2 to 3 hours. Keep it in the basin and cut as required.

Mince with scrambled egg
Any kind of meat may be used for the mince. Put 1lb mince in saucepan with ½ pint stock and 2 cups of stale wholemeal bread crumbs. Mix well and warm just slightly. Add two lightly scrambled eggs to the mixture.

10 Dobermanns Around the World

There is an International Dobermann Club and, in addition to the countries listed in this chapter, the following countries are members: Belgium, Republic of Ghana, Denmark, Germany, Finland, Italy, Luxembourg, Norway, Austria, Portugal, Sweden and Spain.

The International Dobermann Club

The first IDC was founded in 1959. The famous German breeder, the late Mr E. Wilking (Von Forell Kennels), and Professor A. Wilhelm from France called for the meeting. About seventeen delegates who represented their countries participated. However, after debates this organisation ceased activities.

In 1978 delegates from eighteen countries re-established the IDC in Munich. The IDC arrange an annual show and IDC champion titles are awarded. Working awards are also given. There is a special IDC show in the Scandinavian countries. The president of the IDC is always the President of the Dobermann Club of Germany.

Puerto Rico

In 1959–60 the first Dobermann arrived in Puerto Rico brought in by the late Jose Alfaro. Alexis Rodriguez brought Dobermanns from the States from the 'Kay Hills' kennels making the breed popular in Puerto Rico.

There are only two all breed clubs in Puerto Rico. The Puerto Rican Kennel Club that is for American points and the F.C.I. which is for P.R. International points.

For the F.C.I. Dobermanns come from Santo Domingo, Venezuela, Canada and United States as well as other countries. The

F.C.I. is registered in Belgica. The club name is 'Federacion Canofila de Puerto Rica'. There are only five Dobermanns who have become Champions in Puerto Rico:

PR.CH. Von Schumamm Babalin (male)
PR.CH. Blackjax Ace of Spades (male)
Dom ven B.I.S. Magesil's Black Octopus CD (AM. pointed) (male)
Dom Magesil's Princess India (female)
PR.CH.Dom Targas Victoria Regina (female)

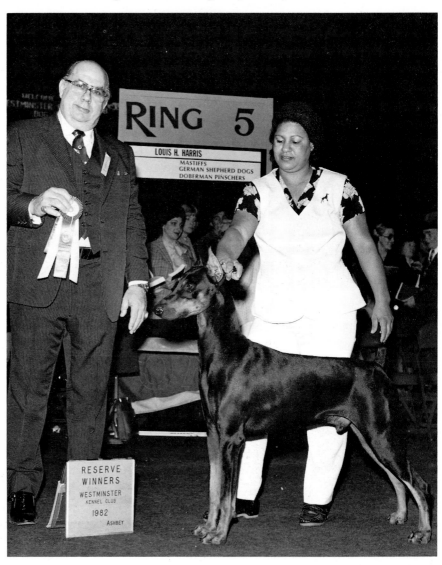

Am Ch Magesils Black Octopus Puerto Rico. Owner Joan Santiago George. Breeder Madeleine George.

Magesil's Black Octopus at only 15 months won Best in Show in Venezuala becoming a Venezualan Champion after two weeks. He became Dominican Champion and then went on to one of the biggest shows in the history of The Westminster Show in 1982 to win Reserve Winner Dog. He is the most outstanding Dobermann in Puerto Rico.

Madeline George is the Founder of the Puerto Rican Dobermann Club which has 53 members.

Switzerland

The Swiss Dobermann Club was founded in 1902 and has belonged to the Swiss Kennel Club since 1909. The Club is divided into nine local clubs, Basle, Berne, Geneva, Jura, Lausanne, Lucerne, Mittelland, Ticino and Zurich. At the present time there are 550 members. The important decisions of the club are made by the delegate conference (1 delegate per 15 local club members plus the members of the Executive Board – 7 people), which takes place once a year in the spring. The club has very strict rules concerning breeding. To breed Dobermanns with pedigrees, stud dog and bitch must pass special tests organised by the club. In the first test (six to twelve month old dogs) the Dobermann is tested in a peaceful situation. In the second test (after fifteen months of age) in a threatening situation. If the dog passes both tests he will be examined by a person qualified to judge Dobermanns in Swiss Dog Shows. This examination is based on the Dobermann Standard deposited with the F.C.I.

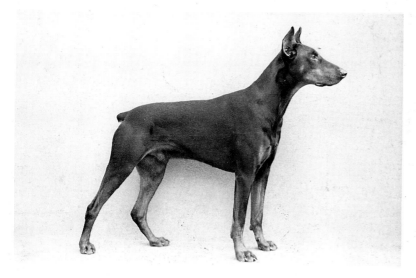

Varo vom Spessart, born 11.9.1971. Owner M. Grunig. Switzerland's most successful Dobermann within the last 15 years.

During 1984 five breeding tests (all three parts) were organised and only nine Dobermanns passed all three parts. Twenty-three dogs were admitted for the tests. An appeal may be filed within fourteen days and then two other judges will judge the dog. The chance to win an appeal is practically nil as the judges are considered very good.

The club prescribes that only dogs older than eighteen months but not older than eight years (an exception is possible for studs) shall be used for breeding. The Swiss allow only one litter per bitch per calendar year and only eight puppies per litter. The puppies must not be sold before they are ten weeks old. They have to be vaccinated and wormed. The buyer receives a pedigree from the breeder of the pups. The Swiss Kennel Club upon application from the Swiss Dobermann Club will issue the documents. The Federal Act for the Protection of Animals (valid after 1 July 1981) forbids the cutting of ears.

Twelve breeders had 21 litters with 109 puppies in 1984. This of course only refers to breeders producing puppies with pedigrees not the 'wild' breeders. Thirty-one Dobermanns were imported and registered with the Swiss Club's Stud Book during the year.

Varo Von Spessart shown in the photograph belonged to an officer of the Bernese Cantonal Police Force. He was the most successful Dobermann in Switzerland within the last fifteen years and had many successes during police duty and rescued many people after the big earthquake in Becurest in 1977.

France

The beginning of the twentieth century saw the Dobermann breed established in Alsace. The dogs had initially come from Germany.

On 13 October 1913 the local association was founded. Interrupted by World War I, the association soon started to grow again when it was re-established in the 1920s and in 1923 it became known as the Dobermann Club of France. The Club was again interrupted by World War II but it now has a membership of two thousand three hundred and has the best breeding record in Europe.

For the last twelve years regular shows under The Central Dog Society have taken place. There have been more than three hundred and fifty entries, with winners being awarded the title 'champions of France'.

There is a National series of tests of dogs' abilities. This plus marks for 'looks' ensure good breeding standards.

There are more and more competitions of all sorts. A 'Working Class' Trials takes place every two years. There are National Civil Defence, Civil Safety competitions which lead to Dobermanns qualifying as e.g. Snow search dogs, Rescue dogs etc.

The Dobermann Club of France belongs to the IDC (International Dobermann Club). The annual show of the IDC leads to the title Champion of the IDC.

Holland

The first Dobermann presented at a Dutch dog show was Troll v Thuringen in 1901. This dog was bred by Otto Göller, the famous Dobermann breeder from the early days. The first litter in Holland was bred by Mr Hof in the Hague in January 1903. Sire of the litter was Erbgraf von Thüringen and the dam was Gutta von Thüringen. This first Dutch litter was obviously a good one because these dogs gained several high places under German judges.

Until the outbreak of World War I in 1914 the best known kennels in Holland were v. Grammont owned by Mr H. Klöppel; v.d. Koningstad owned by Mr C.L.v.Akkeren; and Rival owned by Mr A. v.d.Schoot. During and after World War I, Holland was very important for the Dobermann breed because due to bad circumstances in Germany very many Dobermanns had died during the war. Many Dobermanns were exported back to Germany and also to the USA; the Dutch Dobermanns of those days were imported to build up the breed in America. Nowadays the breeding of Dobermanns in Holland is still on a very high level.

Dutch Dobermanns often win the big titles and prizes at the important shows in Germany. Dutch Dobermanns are exported all over the world these days.

The well known Dutch Kennels are (in alphabetical order) v.Franckenhorst, v.Georgstolz, v.Neerlands Stam, v.'t Smeulveen, v.Stevinhage.

Holland is a member of the International Dobermann Club which had been 'sleeping' for several years and was 'brought back to life' in 1978. The first IDC Winners Show 'new style' was held in Strassbourg in 1979. The 1983 show was held in Holland. The 1984 show in Italy and the 1985 show will be held in Spain.

Indonesia

Until the Dobermann Club of Indonesia was formed in 1981 no regular Dobermann shows were held. From then on there are now about four Specialty shows and one or two All Breed Shows in one year.

To become an Indonesian Champion one needs to have three Challenge Certificates (for Indonesian local breed) and four Challenge Certificates for imports (one of which must be a major Challenge Certificate or Best of Breed or Best Opposite Sex) under different judges.

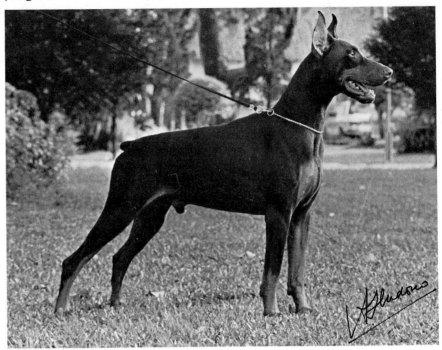

Indonesian Ch Moonbeam's Showboat. Owners Dr Andi Hudono, Hendra Gunawan and Dedy Tjahjono. The No 1 Dobermann in Indonesia in 1984.

Up until early 1985 there are only seven Indonesian Champions. All the judges come from abroad.

The Dobermann has existed in Indonesia since the 1950s but not until 1976 when there were some fresh imports did the Dobermann start to become popular. There were some American, Japanese German Dutch and Australian imports that have become the foundation stock of the Indonesian Dobermann.

The Indonesian Dobermann Club also belongs to the International Dobermann Club.

Japan

The history of the Dobermann in Japan officially goes back to the record of an import Junker o Butersburg of Lux o.d. Blankenburg descent from German in 1929.

Japan has seen the prosperity of the Dobermann since 1941, and the end of the Second World War. The dogs that brought about the popularity of the breed were the dogs from Europe – there were very few from the USA.

Though some twenty male and female dogs including Junker Bw. Arko VonderScheffelsburg had been imported for twelve years before the end of the war it is sad that one does not see their descendants. They were forced to retire by other dogs that were imported one after the other. In those days it was mostly German Shepherd dogs that were placed for military or police use and the Dobermann then was kept mostly for family use.

After the war Dobermanns have seen the poor and sad days. The Japanese Police Dog Association was formed in 1947 in place of the Military Dog Association and then we began to see their prosperity. The dogs kept by the American soldiers in Japan took a great part in the improvement and development of the kind as new blood. They made the second start of the history. Since then Allan o Fürstenfeld, Emir von der Freisenberg, and others have been imported from German and contributed to the great development of the Dobermann. Especially famous is Lex v Forell who made a new epoch in the history and is regarded as the basis of the modern Dobermanns in Japan.

Besides Flint, Bodo, Rondo Odin and others were imported from the Forell Kennel in Germany and all contributed to the Japan Dobermann world. From America a lot of good dogs were imported including Sebastian von Graefe, Karellmar's Kenbric, and Karellmar's Marc Sangstar who took an active part in breeding. From England came Ch Tahase Sormy D Destar in 1965, and Bonby Dutch Dictator was recently imported. The Japanese have been fortunate in that they have excellent dogs from mixing the blood of American and German dogs. Recently the number of dogs from America appears to be larger than those from Germany.

The Japanese Dobermann Club is aiming to heighten the standard of Japanese dogs by mixing good points of both American and German. The Club belongs to the International Dobermann Club and the system for judging show, obedience and working competitions is the German one.

At the Japan Championship Show there were two hundred and seventy Dobermanns in 1984 and one thousand at the Japan Training Competition.

Israel

It is difficult to say when Dobermanns were first seen in Israel but it is believed to have been around 1940. In the second half of the 1940s

Mr Manfred Josephs joined the police force and he trained Dobermanns and was a top breeder who was highly respected by his fellow breeders.

The Israel Dobermann Club (IDC) was founded in 1973 by a group of Dobermann enthusiasts. The club is affiliated to the Israel Kennel Club (IKC) and the IKC is a member of the Federation Cynologique Internationale (FCI).

The Israel Dobermann club follows the German system for breeding. Every litter is checked by the Breed Warden and IKC issues pedigrees only after the approval of the Breed Warden. The Club has Breeding Eligibility Tests which consist of three tests. 1 Confirmation, 2 Temperament, 3 Hip Dysplasia results. The aim for these tests is to eliminate all unsuitable material for breeding. Pedigrees are issued only to puppies whose parents have the above tests.

The Israel Dobermann club holds shows, produces a special magazine and has Schutzhund training. In 1977, 1022 Dobermann puppies were born.

USA

The first Dobermann (or Doberman as it is spelt in America) registered in the USA was recorded with the American Kennel Club in the back of the 1908 Stud Register under Foreign Dogs. A black male, Doberman Intelectus # 122650 was whelped 20 June 1908 out of import parents. The first American Bred (and first male) to win an American Championship was CH.Dobermann Dix in 1912. Dobes were becoming popular as early as 1901, the DPCA first being listed as a Specialty Club in 1913, and officially recognized in 1919.

In 1921 many imports were arriving as the breed had recovered in Germany from World War I and over the next fifteen years many top German dogs came to America, among them the dog Lux vd Blankenburg, imported by Glen Staines, Ponchartrain Kennels in 1927, who sired six Sieger and Siegeren titles and nineteen American champions. Over half of the American champions between 1946 and 1950 traced a direct line to Lux. The most outstanding bitch imported was Jessy vd Sonnenhoehe who had been Best at two successive Sieger shows and produced a Sieger and a Siegeren in Germany. In America, she produced thirteen Champions in only two breedings.

The advent of World War II ceased importations. Much of the Modern 'Show' popularity of Dobermanns was due to the influence of Peggy Adamson's Damasyn line, particularly the most successful show dog and sire CH Dictator v Glenhugel. 'Tator' sired fifty-two champions and many of today's top breeders base their lines on him.

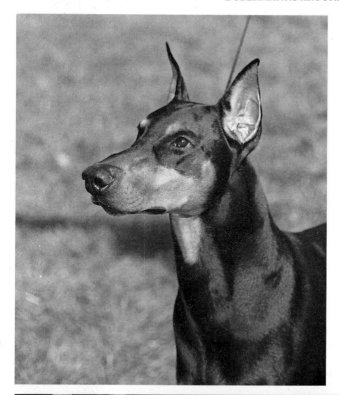

Am Ch Renejade
The Jazz Singer.
Owner Nancy
Christensen.

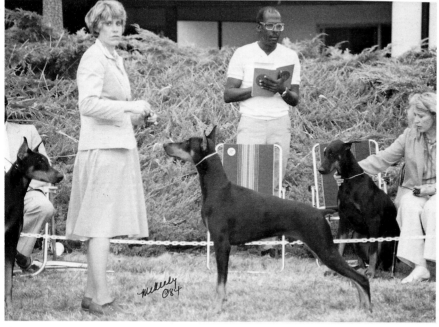

Alpha Omega's
Mister Trooper
USA. Owner Nancy
Christensen.

Other top foundation kennels during the 40s and 50s included Rancho Dobes who produced the outstanding CH Rancho Dobes Storm, along with many other very good champions. Tess Hensler's Ahrtal name is still a winner today, after over seventy home-bred champions. Ahrtals foundation bitch, Meadowmist Isis of Ahrtal produced a total of thirty-five puppies, with seventeen becoming champions. Of the many top winning and producing dogs were CH Felix v Ahrtal (blue) who produced twenty-eight champions, and his black brother CH Florian sired fourteen. CH Cassio v Ahrtal another black sired thirty-seven champions. Many of today's breeders have their foundation in the Ahrtal line.

Jack and Eleanor Brown had many champions and are also behind many of today's winners. Their CH Browns Eric sired twenty-eight champions, CH Browns Dion sired thirty-five Champions and CH. Browns B Brian twice won Best of Breed at the DPCA National Specialty and the Stud Dog class at that show three times.

Marks Tey The Saint USA. Breeder Joanna Walker.

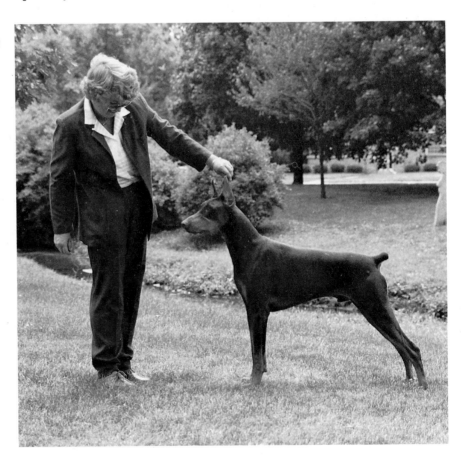

Joanna Walker's Marks Tey prefix has greatly influenced the breed, for Joanna's work in writing and working with Rescue and Pilot dogs has been tremendous. Her best known champions and producers include CH Marks Tey Melanie who was the dam of eight and grand dam of thirty-seven champions, CH Derek of Marks Tey sire of ten champions, CH Marks Tey Shawn CD, sire of sixteen Champions and the famous CH Marks Tey The Maverick who only sired two champions, both of whom have gone on to sire champions and champion producers (CH Silent Sentrys Marauder WAC and CH Mesmerol Bari of Marks Tey CD ROM). The true measure of Maverick's fame was that his life was ended, at the height of an illustrious show career with a bullet sustained while saving a family member from a mugging in Chicago. A true Dobermann!!

Joanna Walker is disturbed that the popularity of the Dobermann has not been in the best interests of the breed and she believes that Pit Bull Terriers and Dobermanns are probably the most abused dogs of any breed, mainly because people get them for the wrong reasons, such as dog fighting, which is illegal, or to enhance the owner's macho image. Although Joanna occasionally raises a litter of top quality show puppies she spends most of her time rescuing mis-treated Dobermanns and training some of them as guide dogs. She has spent time at Pilot Dogs Inc. in order to gain far more experience in training lead dogs for the blind. Pilot Dogs Inc. is a non-profit organisation, founded in 1950. What is so wonderful about this scheme is that the blind person is not only given a trained dog free of charge, but receives his transportation, meals and lodging for the entire month he spends in Ohio working with his dog.

Joanna has had six Dobermanns which she has rescued from appaling conditions of cruelty that have graduated to become guide dogs for the blind because all the attention must be devoted to their master – the tremendous amount of work and concentration to achieve this in a Dobermann is really extraordinary.

Pilot dogs, in addition to having dogs donated also raises its own puppies in a breeding programme. Pilot Dogs is the only guide dog organisation in the USA which accepts Dobermanns with the qualification that they must not measure more than 25″ (.6 m) from floor to shoulder, as the dogs must be small enough not to take up too much room when acccompanying their owner in cars and buses.

Just as not every dog is suitable to become a guide dog so every blind person is not automatically a suitable candidate. For Joanna Walker the idea of using abandoned dogs to train as guide dogs for the blind has provided a tremendous satisfaction at a not inconsiderable cost, paying for the spaying of each animal and also the cost of shipping them from Centralia, Illinois to Columbus for training. It is very hard parting with the dogs but the sadness of separation is tempered by the fact that she knows the dogs will be loved as few pets are loved and will be sharing one of the closest relationships that can exist between man and animal.

Jane Kay's outstanding CH Kay Hills Paint the Town Red produced twelve champions including CH Kay Hills Witch Soubretta who produced eighteen champions and this is still the record for most champions produced by any American Dobermann Bitch.

One of the first smooth elegant modern Dobermanns of importance was CH Singenwalds Prince Kuhio, who sired thirty-six champions. Adding to the smooth modern look was Ted Links CH Tedell Eleventh Hour, who at eight months old was the youngest Dobermann ever to go best in Show at an all breed event and who sired fourteen champions.

CH Dolph v Tannenwald and CH Gra Lemor Demetrius vd Victor were both top winners as well as top sires.

In the early 70s Mary Rodger's CH Marienburg Sun Hawk began winning and went on to be a top producer with over sixty champions to his credit and with more likely to come as he has been dead only a few years. Marienburg, among many winners, also is known for the beautiful CH Marienburg Mary Hartman who won the DPCA Speciality once as a young Special then returned to win from the veterans class.

CH Andelanes Indigo Rock was the winner of twenty-four all breeds Bests in Show and the sire of sixteen champions including two Best in Show daughters. Rocky is the foundation for Do Dillon McLaughlins Rocado prefix which has in a few years finished six champions and campaigned the Rock grandson CH Renejade the Jazz Singer to top winning status. The Jazz Singer's sire, CH Bishops Borong v Rock, owned by Do Dillon Mclaughlin sired eleven champions out of forty-four puppies.

Another top modern sire was CH Highland Satan's Image who produced forty-four champions.

Only time will tell if the current Dobermann winners will measure up. However, the number one Dobermann for the past four consecutive years CH Eagles Devil D, is showing much promise as a sire with several champions and others pointed. Other top winners promising to be good sires include CH Pajants Encore v Rockelle, CH Cabras Dark and Debonaire, CH Renejade the Jazz Singer and CH Arco Dob Mann.

In America, much status is based on the various ranking systems. Each counts a different set of points for other dogs defeated in Breed, Group and Best in Show competition. The most prestigious ranking is probably that of the DPCA which allots one point for each dog in competition in Best of Breed only. As an example, 78 in competition, BOB winner is awarded 78 points. These totals are kept through the year according to the American Kennel Gazette reports and the Top Twenty Elite are invited to compete in a unique event at the National DPC Specialty each year.

This Top twenty event was created by a group of people who wanted an extra special competition, where each dog could be evaluated using a scale of points based on the standard so that no one fault or virtue could be allowed to dominate, and where each dog could be allowed a much longer period of time for the evaluation – time for the judge to think and recheck each animal – time for the spectator to really see each one. In this competition three judges are selected, secretly, and no one but the committee knows until the day of the show who is judging. One judge is to be a breeder of renown, one a professional handler of Dobermanns, one an all breed judge. The event itself is set up to be a showcase of what we refer to as the cream of the crop and each winner a lasting credit to the breed. Regardless of the outcome, it is quite an event to see.

11 Veterinary Care

Allergy

A very methodical approach is needed to eliminate gradually those chemicals and proteins (allergens) present in the dog's food and general environment which seem to cause it to suffer from hot itchy skin, scurfy dry coat and sometimes ear problems. These are some of the signs of hypersensitivity brought about by long or short exposure times (sensitization) often to more than one allergy.

An allergic reaction may be a delayed one with a long sensitizing time as for house dust and house dust mites or it may be immediate as in a wasp sting. A whole body reaction to a sting may rapidly lead to shock and must be presented to your vet.

Long term skin itchiness (pruritus) can be complicated by self-inflicted injury (chewing or scratching).

Testing for allergic reactions commonly shows up fleas, food colourings, house dust and house dust mites.

Anaemia

A reduction in exercise tolerance, with pallor of the membranes in the mouth, may be due to anaemia which shows as a reduction in the oxygen carrying ability of the blood. This anaemia may itself be due to a lack of minerals and vitamins reaching the dog's blood-forming tissues. It may also be due to recent or continuing blood loss, blood-borne parasites, or heavy internal or external parasites (for example hookworm, severe flea problems), rarely is it due to poisons. A blood sample often helps to build up a general picture and helps monitor the effect of supportive therapy.

Anal glands

The symptoms of problems are that the dog continually smells of a foetid, musky odour. The dog frequently rubs its bottom on the ground. Anal glands are part of a dog's olfactory identity, as we often know too well. The passage of normal motions will help express the contents of these glands as well as the cleaning that some dogs give themselves.

When the tiny ducts (which open into the anus) become blocked the glands will get more and more full, become very uncomfortable (causing 'scooting') as well as displacement biting of the tail and legs and can become very infected and hot. Anal gland abscesses are very painful and should receive veterinary attention. Fortunately the breed does not appear to be troubled significantly by this problem. Special dietary roughage sprinkled on food daily will supply extra fibre, lack of which contributes to this problem.

Arthritis

This term means inflammation of a joint – in an acute case, redness, heat, pain and swelling with reluctance to use the affected limb (i.e. lame). Sometimes this process goes on gradually inside the joint (limbs or spine) over a long time and the dog goes lame sometime after the arthritic change has started.

Numbered amongst the causes are poor body conformation, more specifically, poor joint development, a sequel to injuries, excessive stress/wear and tear on a joint and sometimes infections, when more than one joint may be involved.

As a first aid measure, paracetamol may be used as an analgesic but your vet would prefer to examine the dog should pain be severe, or prolonged.

One of the first steps to ease lameness is to hose or cold poultice a joint, with little or no exercise and a supporting crepe bandage. To further the diagnosis, radiographs may be necessary.

Bacteria, viruses and the skin

Impetigo or multiple focal infections of the skin may be seen as a result of direct bacterial entry on ventral abdominal skin (red spots, pus-capped). 'Chin spots' started by the mites are complicated by secondary bacterial infection which justifies antibiotic and antiparasite therapy and so allows the skin to re-establish a new balance with the mites. Larger areas of skin can become invaded by bacteria especially in thickened oozing skin lesions called wet eczema, usually self inflicted and in a vicious circle of itch/scratch (fleas, anal glands?)

Any damage into deeper skin layers can lead to bacterial entry.

Seborrhoea is a skin condition where excess oil comes to the skin surface. It is a secondary result from internal disorders. Here bacteria and fungi grow in the grease and produce a musky, dank smell. Supplementation and correction to the diet will effect a cure but shampoos (with conditioning; or coal tar and sulphur) give temporary relief. Both viruses and bacteria when causing systemic disease lead to changes in the skin or coat (dull, staring, dry ...) Warts are often viral-induced and appear more commonly on older dogs and these can be treated by your vet.

SKIN TUMOURS

As opposed to skin-gland cysts, genuine skin tumours are rare. Anal adenomata are problems in older dogs and are thought to arise from the skin glands. Multiple, enlarging, skin thickenings, in older dogs ought to be checked by your vet with a view to biopsy.

TUMOURS BENEATH THE SKIN

These range from enveloped fatty growths (lipomas) to mammary tumours. As much as the thought of cancer is distressing it is much wiser to allow your vet to make an early examination and decide on appropriate action than allow a mammary growth to spread along the abdomen or to grow so large that it ulcerates the skin and the size jeopardises good skin closure after surgical removal of the affected area. Also, rapidly growing tumours can send seed tumours in the blood into the lungs where secondary growths develop. It may be that you will be put at ease by the diagnosis made at the time of examination, or after consenting to a biopsy.

Balanitis

Some discharge, yellow or off-white may be seen occasionally on the penis of the dog. Persistent and larger amounts with constant licking of the yellow to green discharge often indicates a balanitis or infection of the sheath, possibly with erosion of the penis and ascending infection.

Any matted hair should be carefully clipped away and the whole area washed with weak peroxide or hypochlorite (Milton) especially inside the sheath. Should blood or ulcerated areas be seen, then professional attention will be necessary. After washing apply soothing antibiotic creams.

On a related subject, a dog may 'spot' blood when sexually excited – this is uncommon but not unknown. Severe infections of the urinary tract will generate blood and pus but other signs of dysuria – such as straining, discomfort and repetition – will be present.

Burns

When chemical burns are suspected, the area should be thoroughly rinsed with a stream of tepid water. If acidic, bicarbonate solution can be added to neutralise and prevent further corrosion. As with heat burns including fat, cold poulticing will greatly reduce the subsequent inflammation. Bland soothing lanolin-based ointment may be used and the area protected from licking.

After such first aid, your dog should be professionally examined whenever there is any cause for concern – especially where a large area of skin is involved (damaged cells release chemicals which *can* cause profound shock) and loss of skin allows serum to ooze with bacteria gaining entry into the body.

Electric burns often involve the mouth. A special acidic cream with "Aspirin" in it is available from your veterinary surgeon to promote painless healing.

Capped elbows

These are areas of thickened skin formed as a result of compression of the skin between underlying bone and hard floor/bed surfaces. Such 'pressure sores' are seen commonly on the elbows and are often rough and scaley to the touch. No infection is usually present. Try to stop your dog from lying on concrete (especially if new), hard floors and beds and use blankets, sponge or deep pile dog bedding. Lanolin, vaseline or talc can be rubbed in to prevent cracking of these areas.

Cardiac disease

See under breed-related diseases on page 113.

Chin spots

These can be treated quite successfully with a solution of peroxide diluted to 5% and dabbed on the spots.

Coughs

A large group of problems ranging from tooth scale and gingivitis through tonsilitis, pharyngitis, laryngitis, tracheitis to congestion and fluid in the lungs. The latter is often seen as a result of poor lung circulation. Of note but of variable annual importance is the clinical syndrome known as infectious laryngo-tracheitis or 'Kennel Cough' for which several vaccines are available. This involves much unproductive coughing (some dirty coloured mucus), retching, lethargy and a mild to moderate fever. Benylin may be useful alone (every 3 to 4 hours) in such cases. Gravity may assist with mucus removal – putting the dog's head and chest lower than its abdomen when it is coughing, but with such signs professional help should be sought. Owing to the infectious nature of the disease your vet may wish to see you separately from the other dogs in the surgery waiting room. A connection with kennels or recently kennelled dogs is not always necessary since the organisms involved may already be present in the dog's airways waiting for some stress factors to overcome the dog's natural defences.

Violent coughing can arise from inhaled foreign bodies (with violent sneezing), from the eating of coarse grass, bone fragments or wood. Agitated behaviour, gagging, dribbling and mouth pawing accompany a piece of bone lodged between the teeth or in the throat. Rapid, calm but firm action is necessary to identify the problem (open weave bandage under top and above lower jaws to pull apart) and your vet should be phoned.

The dry heart cough should also be brought to the attention of your vet.

Constipation

This is fortunately not a common problem. It may follow diarrhoea, the eating of bones or where there is insufficient roughage in the diet. Extra fibre in the form of cooked vegetables, bran or a proprietary product can be added or the use of senna pod extracts and liquid paraffin in more difficult cases.

In the entire dog, an enlarged prostate may lead to reluctance to defaecate and secondary constipation. Sometimes, long term constipation and straining can lead to a pocket forming in the rectum (requiring manual emptying) and also a perineal lesion (hernia). Difficulty in defaecating any longer than two or three days must receive attention.

Cystitis

Cystitis is an inflammation of the bladder more commonly seen in bitches. Repetitive straining and discomfort are a feature. Blood, mucus with pus as well as discoloured urine may be seen with irritating bladder stones and also with prostatic infection in the dog. Unusually, indoor urination may take place involuntarily as the inflammed bladder is thicker walled and is too painful to stretch with a normal amount of urine.

The first step after contacting your vet is to collect a urine sample. One way is to adapt an old coat hanger or a long piece of stout wire as a handle and holder for a long flat clean pie dish. This can be decanted into a clean herb or jam jar which has been thoroughly rinsed out with boiling water to remove any traces of sugar. Clean samples may be left in a cool place or in the fridge overnight if necessary so long as the veterinary surgery receives the samples early the next day.

Persistent haematuria (blood) and dysuria may require radiography, including the use of contrast techniques.

Diarrhoea

Severe, prolonged loose motions with straining, sometimes with blood, lead to the associated problem of dehydration (the body deprived of adequate water for blood and tissues). This type of diarrhoea can quickly turn into an enteritis, even a gastro-enteritis, if not checked by kaolin, kaolin and morphine, glucose-water on a little-and-often basis and starvation.

Simple diarrhoea may be checked by a restricted quantity of light diet and boiled glucose water (one rounded dessert spoon per pint). A normal motion may have a loose end but straining is not usually a feature. When straining and blood or foetid smell are present, a professional visit is necessary. Personal hygiene of both the dog and yourself is important.

In pups, diarrhoea may also be the result of too much milk, chewed up wood, too much to eat and, occasionally, roundworms. In adult dogs, although a rare problem, regularly loose motions passed several (5 to 7) times daily with no straining could indicate an inability to digest or absorb the food eaten. Weight loss and pronounced ribs are a feature of pancreatic insufficiency. A faeces sample can be analysed by a veterinary practice laboratory to assess this problem.

Diarrhoea can also be a problem when excessive quantities of fluids are being drunk - this is usually coupled with increased urination. A sample of urine plus a consultation should be considered to find out the reason for excessive thirst.

Dewclaws removal and tail docking

I am sure that these two subjects cause much concern to both owners and veterinary surgeons when regarding puppies' welfare. The clearly defined breed standards are being made more open to informed veterinary opinion as we work to put the puppies' present and future welfare considerations first.

As these moves are being made, I would consider it best that a skilful and understanding veterinary surgeon undertakes what is undeniably a mutilation of puppies under his care preferably by thermocautery at 3 to 4 days of age at a special appointment.

The ear

Regular examination, by sight and smell, of your dog's ears is another way to care for your pet.

EXCESS WAX

Any noticeable wax or yeasty, musty smell must lead you to use bland basic ear cleaning liquids such as olive oil, liquid paraffin, baby oil or proprietary wax solvents from your vet. Excess wax accumulation can rapidly lead to over growth of yeasts and certain bacteria, erosion and bleeding, infection and pus with liquid pus/wax and a very unpleasant smell. Fortunately, in our breed, the open nature of the ears allows easy hygiene and good air circulation.

EAR MITES

Rarely in the dog does the ear mite Otodectes cause a primary otitis, but one mite present is one too many for most dogs – although many can be seen amongst ear wax in young puppies. Attention to wax removal and up to 30 days insecticidal ear drops will remove the problem. Regular checking is part of the general health care for your dog.

UNCOMPLICATED EXCESS WAX

Excessive wax build-up without a primary cause (muddy water, ear mites etc) also needs regular care. You may have heard of dogs that have waxy ears which have been neglected so much that yeasts and other undesirable bacteria turn the accumulated wax into liquid pus. Then there is the very real danger of middle and inner ear disease as the ear drum becomes damaged.

AURAL HAEMATOMA

This may arise from a foreign body in the ear, or excess wax with/ without ear mites. The swelling is a result of whiplash damage to blood vessels in the ear flap caused by excessive shaking and scratching of the ears. A large pool of blood collects, usually separating the skin from the inner cartilage until the enclosed pressure equals that of escaping blood and is thus self-limiting. For that reason it is inadvisable to drain the swelling immediately but to give the damaged blood vessels time to seal and then a few days later drain and surgically apply a spongy pressure pad plus special dressings. Undrained and untreated small haematomas may not lead to any distortion of the ear flap but larger ones do lead to 'cauliflower' ears. Primary causes must be treated.

SPLITS

Splits in the ear flap bleed profusely and result from fighting or hedge/barbed-wire damage. A special bandage and haemostatic measures will normally sort these out without requiring surgery.

Elizabethan Collar

A useful device when treating a dog for cuts or wounds with stitches, to prevent the animal from biting and aggravating the condition.

Some vets keep this in the surgery for people to borrow. They are simple to make however, by cutting out the bottom of a plastic bucket which the head goes through. Punch four or more holes around this hole, thread some string through these holes and fasten to dog's collar.

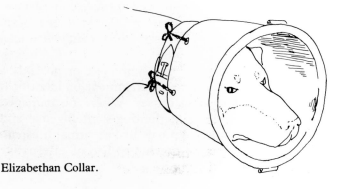

Elizabethan Collar.

The open end must be sufficiently far away from the nose to prevent licking and may present problems when feeding. If this is the case, then remove briefly to allow eating and drinking, or raise the bowl on a block of wood.

The collar may sound and even look awful but most dogs after the first few minutes accept them quite well.

Epilepsy

As will be brought out in the section on homeopathic medicine, this subject covers such a diversity of causes that, where conventional medicine alters a dog's alertness and behaviour, or possibly even increases fit frequency, I feel that alternative medical treatment should be explored since it involves the whole of the dog's body, character and background.

A fit usually lasts only a short time and involves pacing, restlessness, total disorientation, unconsciousness, often involuntary urination and defaecation with alternating or continuous muscular movements, often with a sudden urge to eat after returning to awareness of its surroundings. The fit may lead into another and can start from sleep or relaxation or even from puppy teething.

Conventional medicine recognises causes originating in the brain and nervous system, ranging from direct trauma at birth, congenital weaknesses such as internal brain fluid accumulation (hydrocephalus) through to certain poisons (like slug bait) and idiosyncratic reactions to anthelmintics, tumours in the older dog and encephalitis as in canine distemper. This leads to the causes outside the central nervous system – since viruses and bacteria enter the body elsewhere before causing fever and toxaemia or direct infection of the brain. Teething and worm infestation may overstimulate the brain via peripheral nerves. It is also possible that diabetes mellitus can cause convulsions. Factors leading to temporary loss of supply of oxygen to the brain such as a difficult birth, cardiac arrest or heart defects may also lead to fits.

It is generally understood that a fit is one sign alone or possibly a group of signs requiring either symptomatic treatment or identification and treatment of the predisposing causes. Where no damaged tissue or growth is present in the brain, the dog's intelligence and personality does not change and many animals live a normal lifespan. In order to help your vet to narrow down the list of alternative diagnoses the following information is useful.

1   Present age, sex (?oestrus) or how old when the first fit occurred?
2   Was this fit the first fit as far as is known (kennelled outside?)
3   When did the event occur–dog asleep/relaxed/sudden excitement/ exercise?
4   Any litter mates or several in-contact dogs affected?
5   Jot down what happened during and after the event and the dog's behaviour after returning to apparent normality.
6   Any relevant background information especially related to possible head injury.
7   Was the dog apparently healthy before the fit or had it had a recent infection?
8   Have any poisons been used in the home, or garden or has the dog strayed into sprayed fields or road verges? Has any old paint, lino or lead toys been chewed?

Should a fit happen to your dog, stay calm, talk and steady the dog through it and try to relax him, when he comes back to awareness. Telephone your vet immediately if you are suspicious that a second fit is going to follow.

Eyes

Common eye problems are due to local irritant splashes, dust or pollen, local injury, the ingrowing eyelash or foreign body. These lead to excess tear production, a reluctance to open the eye much in strong light, conjunctivitis and sometimes swollen eyelids. Cold compresses or irrigation with witch-hazel solutions, using tepid water may bring relief. Any injury to the cornea, or conjunctivitis persisting for more than 24 to 36 hours, should be referred for examination as they could indicate a more serious local or general problem.

False pregnancy

Here, a bitch may behave as if she was truly pregnant – variable often increased appetite, enlarged reddened teats, enlarged abdomen, 'soft' behaviour and sometimes 'nest making' and 'toy guarding' up to 9 to 10 weeks from mid season. Lactation may begin.

Should her behaviour be very depressed or the nest making unreasonable, your vet can inject or prescribe hormone tablets that will not interfere with future breeding plans. Your vet may only advise if your bitch is comfortable, but may give you diuretic tablets to ease the milk pressure and ask you to check regularly the mammary glands for any of the hot painful and bright to mottled red signs of mastitis. Homoeopathic treatment is also very useful here.

Painless, hard saucer-like swellings are often seen and these sometimes join up to form one long swelling on one or both sides. Hot and cold compresses may make your bitch more comfortable.

Fish Hook

This diagram shows the correct way of removing a fish hook.

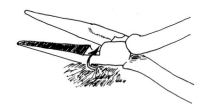

Removing a fish
hook.

Flatulence

This is an individual dog's problem normally dependent on diet (tinned/fresh meat, complete food diet, excess or lack of dietary fibre). Careful alteration of the diet to less potent food is needed with balanced roughage playing its part in reducing the level of fermentable food still able to reach the large bowel. Digestive enzyme deficiencies as in pancreatic insufficiency, or poor bile flow can also lead to secondary large intestine fermentation. Food containing carbon (e.g. burnt toast, activated charcoal) can reduce these odours, which can be complemented by anal gland secretions.

Fleas and flies

It may be said that fleas do not respect pedigrees. They cause a lot of irritation and also create allergic reactions leading to self-inflicted wounds. Check your dog during grooming for the dark mahogany flea that slips through the hair, or the gritty dark flea dirts picked up by the flea comb.

Take action using flea sprays/powder and shampoos and don't forget the bedding, favourite chair and the carpets (household flea sprays/powder are available and frequent hoovering helps since these long lived fleas and their eggs are present there).

Flies must not be forgotten – it is very unpleasant to pick maggots from the skin and hair of incontinent or diarrhoeic dogs (especially when kennelled) after blow flies have laid their eggs: it cannot be very pleasant for the dog either since the skin is often badly damaged and sore.

Foot problems

BROKEN NAILS

Usually acute pain, some blood loss and sore. Best treated if 'quick' exposed by local anaesthetic, cutting and cautery. If free of the quick chip carefully as near to start of the split as possible.

CUT PADS

Flap cuts heal with difficulty even when freshly sutured. Deep incised wounds (refer to haemorrhaging) respond to suturing when fresh. Small nicks may be dressed and covered.

THORNS IN PADS

Difficult to find and to squeeze out. Poultice with Epsom Salts or use homoeopathic Silicea.

CYSTS

Rare in breed. Hot Epsom salts poultice.

TAR AND PAINT

Removed with proprietary 'soft gel' hand cleansers, even hot water if paint of suitable type.

OVER STRETCH, SHORT TERM LAMENESS

Cold poulticing and rest. If lameness marked seek professional attention. Paracetamol tablets useful first aid.

GENERAL PENETRATION OF FOREIGN BODIES

Grass seeds, grit, broken-off sticks, glass. Usual to see marked swelling, heat, pain and redness between toes and wrist (carpal), joints or ankle (tarsal) joints. Grass seeds can track up the leg. When the swelling is so marked your vet may wish to give diuretic, antibiotic and anti-inflammatory drugs for a day in order to facilitate explorative procedures. Also of great use is homoeopathic silicea.

Foreign bodies

This type of problem leads us on from the feet to the broader problem of foreign bodies reaching the nasal cavity, eye, ear and stomach or intestine. In all these cases, irritation and abnormal behaviour is observed. Sneezing, tear production, rubbing eyes, constant head shaking and scratching and head tilt, grass eating and retching, small bowel movements with or without diarrhoea respectively may be observed. In my opinion, it is worth trying to induce vomiting when gloves or socks have been swallowed. Several large crystals of washing soda plus warm water will assist the removal. Should several hours or a day have passed before such items are missed, then resort to liquid paraffin and bulky foods (porridge, brown bread) to coat any sharp edges. Stones are a problem as they can lodge and close the gut, but incredibly, quite large stones are first palpated in the large intestine and can be assisted out as just mentioned without surgery.

However, in all cases of foreign bodies, your vet should be involved in their removal at the earliest opportunity since foreign bodies will create unnecessary serious damage if they are simply ignored. The unusual forms of foreign bodies include spring clips from dogs leads (through a toe or round the tendon above the hock joint) and fish hooks. The latter require a local anaesthetic ahead of the barbs which have to be pushed on and be exposed to be cut off before the rest of the hook can be pulled out in the opposite direction.

Gums and general mouth care

Peridontal disease is a condition where tooth roots become exposed to food, saliva and bacteria due to the destructive effect of toothscale on the sensitive gum margins. The gum retracts and the tooth becomes less protected. One effective way to prevent this is to carry out regular descaling of the teeth and to use crisp/hard food for self-cleaning. Where soft scale is present careful wiping with 3% hydrogen peroxide/tooth powder on cotton wool may remove most of the scale – watch the powerful carnassial teeth (!) and wipe/descale. Always work from the gum to tooth tip. Never use sharp wooden/metal devices for scaling unless specially purchased and, if in doubt, consult your veterinary surgeon.

When checking the teeth look for any chips or fractures or discolouration and bring them to your vet's attention at your next routine visit.

Occasionally, lip fold eczema may develop – wiping with 3% peroxide and dabbing dry usually prevents erosion and infection.

Hair loss or alopecia

Hair growth is a complex continuous cycle regulated in part by hormones. The compound hair follicle of the dog contains both a large coarse guard hair from a central follicle together with several soft undercoat hairs from smaller satellite follicles.

After a period of rapid hair growth, the follicle stops producing a new hair for a time. The renewed hair remains in place in the follicle until a new hair is made to grow once more beneath it. The older one is shed in a normally continuous cycle of loss and replacement. Any disturbance in this imbalance will lead to changes in coat texture (more coarse, for example) and in hair replacement (fewer made, giving a thinner, sparse coat or alopecia).

Such disturbances may be due to hormones, allergies, diet (lack of special skin oils, minerals and vitamins) bacterial infection of the general skin (dermatitis) or specifically of the hair follicles. Aging has an effect on the skin and coat. Also involved is the hair loss associated with psychological and idiopathic (no apparent) causes. Parasites (already considered) and a physical injury (burns, scalds, chemicals) also play a part.

Two more recognisable hormone problems involve the thyroid and the ovaries. (Hypo-thyroidism and hyper oestrogenism). A slowed down (hypo-active) thyroid tends to cause lethargy, obesity as well as a sparse and coarse coat. Diagnosis is not always straight forward although blood samples help by measuring a marker hormone and cholesterol levels. Thyroxine therapy usually assists with borderline as well as positive hypo-thyroid cases.

Thyroxine tablets also help to correct the hair loss caused by 'ovarian imbalance' or hyper-oestrogenism, since the body's hormones are always inter-acting. Alopecia is commonly seen in association with the oestrogen peak just prior to true oestrus. Such coat changes are usually only temporary. More continuous oestrogen effects will lead to greater hair loss but this spontaneously cures itself, especially if helped by thyroxine therapy.

Canine Cushing's Syndrome shows as symmetrical hair loss but the pendulous abdomen, excessive thirst, appetite and urination help to differentiate this particular hormone problem.

Bacterial dermatitis with *Demodex* mite/secondary bacterial invasion of hair follicles will lead to direct adverse effects on hair replacement with rapid hair loss but little replacement.

A combination of conventional and homoeopathic treatment should prove successful in these cases - including the use of relevant hormones, plus symptomatic treatment and iodine.

Remember that the skin reflects deeper mental or physical problems than just those seen on the surface and that sometimes the only symptoms of disease of the whole body are skin problems.

Hepatic disease

See under breed-related diseases on page 113.

Infectious diseases

The main diseases of dogs include those caused by the distemper, the infectious hepatitis and the parvo-viruses plus the two types of leptospire bacteria. Also frequently a problem are the respiratory viruses and bacteria, principally the *Bordetella* bacterium and the adeno-and para-influenza viruses. Not to be forgotten is the ever-present risk of tetanus from the *Clostridiumital* bacterium, and the rabies virus for imported dogs.

Briefly, before describing the common signs of such diseases, it is important to stress that vaccines are available for use in protecting your dog.

All batches of vaccines are thoroughly checked before marketing. Also available are specific antisera (containing high levels of the protective proteins called antibodies) to be injected into a dog suffering from the specific disease or into a puppy getting little or no colostrum.

When a puppy is born, it will have been given antibodies by the mother across the placenta and also by the colostrum (first milk). From the colostrum, antibodies are absorbed for only a few hours after birth and after that they can protect the gut by their continued presence there. After an initial high-level protection, blood antibody levels fall in an exponential way and it is generally assumed that for most puppyhood diseases 10 to 12 weeks of age is the danger time – time to become vaccinated to boost an active immunity rather than depend on the fading passive one given by the dam.

Parvo-virus antibodies passively transferred from the mother react with most vaccine parvo-viruses up to the age of 16 to 18 weeks rendering vaccination ineffective until that age. It is becoming increasingly recommended that a final parvo-virus vaccination be given at 18 to 20 weeks of age for a meaningful immunity.

Leptospirosis vaccines contain killed bacteria – they can be given as a course of 2 vaccinations as early as 10 weeks since any antibodies do not interfere too much with the vaccine. Leptospirosis is still a common problem in rats both in town and country. Distemper is less frequently seen but does recur in cities and some urban areas. Canine parvo-virus also flares up in poorly vaccine-responsive or unvaccin-ated dogs and was first seen as a very serious and epizootic disease not many years ago. It is because your dog does not regularly contact 'field' or 'wild' strains of disease that repeated annual vaccination is necessary – the vaccine acts as a regular reminder to your dog's im-mune system so that if a virulent wild strain *is* met the body defences are quick to spot, recognise and eliminate the disease organism. As you will read, all these diseases are serious and prevention is a very important part of caring for your dog.

DISTEMPER

Affects all parts of the body, including the nervous system, digestive system, eyes, lungs and skin. It is also called 'hardpad' since the pads and nose become hardened by extra rough layers of keratin. Fever, lethargy, conjunctivitis (very purulent, spectacled eyelids) coughing, diarrhoea, fits, leg twitching, even paralysis and death, may be seen singly or in a combination. Transmission is via inhalation or ingestion of virus particles from the coughs and sneezes and discharges of in-fected dogs.

INFECTIOUS HEPATITIS

Like distemper, rarely seen thanks to vaccination. The virus mainly affects the liver but also other organs such as the kidney, blood vessel and the eye ('blue eye'). Blood clotting is interfered with also. Thirst, fever, lethargy, vomiting and diarrhoea with blood, colic, swollen inflamed liver (with or without jaundice) and nervous signs with pale-ness/blood splashing in the mouth, may be present but sometimes there is little time for many signs to develop before death occurs. Transmission again is via infective discharges from other dogs' saliva, faeces and urine.

LEPTOSPIROSIS

Leptospira icterohaemorrhagiae is associated mainly with liver disease and jaundice (plus dysentery) and *Leptospira canicola* mainly affecting the kidneys, (mouth and tongue ulcers, uraemia and occasional jaund-ice). Both cause fever, lethargy, vomiting, thirst, and colic. Blood transfusion may be necessary.

It is important to recognise that *Leptospira icterohaemorrhagiae* is a serious Zoonoses (Weil's Disease) and that animals which have re-covered may remain as inapparent carriers of the disease (capable of infecting other dogs themselves but rarely the cat). Transmission is by inhalation or ingestion of freshly voided urine or from the external genitalia of the infected dog. The bacteria can remain in contaminated water for several weeks.

PARVO-VIRUS

Small virus but a very big problem. It grows in actively dividing cells, principally the heart cells of the very young (six week old) pup and the stomach and intestinal cells of older pups and adult dogs. In puppies of under six weeks of age the disease is usually fatal (several dying in a litter suddenly or after a short time of distressed breathing and collapse). Where pups do recover it must be recognised that permanent heart damage may have been caused (exercise intolerance for example).

In older pups and adult dogs, only a small number actually die with proper nursing and veterinary care. This is because the control of continuous vomiting and diarrhoea to reduce shock and dehydration is mostly successful. The diarrhoea is particularly foul-smelling, pink and mixed with blood – and intravenous fluids and nutrients are necessary for several days in order to keep the dog alive. The parvo-virus is very resistant to weather and disinfectants – bleach is the best household disinfectant. It is transmitted via faeces and vomit and indirectly by feet and clothing.

TETANUS

Bacterial toxins are produced by the *Clostridiumital* bacteria typically in closed, dirty puncture wounds (especially those contaminated by horse droppings or in certain soil types). These toxins affect nerve and muscle functions, causing jerky muscle spasms, hypersensitivity to touch, light and noise, protrusion of the third eyelid, erect ears, arched neck and a 'locked jaw'. Routine vaccination is not necessary but it is available, along with antisera.

Tetanus has a slower course than strychnine poisoning but has many signs in common.

VIRAL AND BACTERIAL INFECTIOUS LARYNGO–TRACHEITIS OR KENNEL COUGH

A contagious disease transmitted by the aerosol discharges and thick ropey mucus of repetitively coughing dogs. Often the two types of disease organisms combine to cause a serious condition (even to pleurisy and pneumonia) but either may cause disease alone under suitable circumstances.

Inherited and breed predisposed disease

Special breed-related diseases are outlined below. Where transmission is established to be by breeding, the correct and responsible action to take is to prevent conception even to the extent of spaying or castration. The quality of the breed must be maintained as must individual welfare considerations.

CERVICAL SPONDYLOLITHESIS

The canine wobbler syndrome is possibly inherited as a recessive trait. The majority of spontaneous cases are seen in young dogs. The signs of hind leg ataxia are seen at slow gaits and also when the dog is brought to a sudden halt from the trot. Then it cannot control its hindquarters which sway and collapse (wobble) almost causing a fall. These signs result from a wide variation in deformation and displacement of cervical (neck) vertebrae and an equally variable compression of the spinal cord. As a consequence, long term treatment is by special vertebral decompression and fusion techniques after confirmation of diagnosis by plain and contrast radiography.

NARCOLEPSY

This is an incurable sleep disorder with loss of muscle tone following such excitement as feeding or vigorous play. Loud talk and patting frequently reverses partial attacks (immobile, glassy eyed) which may proceed unchecked to complete collapse.

POLYOSTOTIC FIBROUS DYSPLASIA

A form of bone cyst which is uncommon but most likely to be seen in the Dobermann and possibly inherited as a recessive trait. One or more cavities may be present within one or more affected bones, filled with fibrous tissue bordered by a thinner outer layer of bone. Swelling may be present in the region, occasionally with pain on palpitation. Treatment is possible.

VON WILLEBRAND'S DISEASE

A blood coagulation defect (haemophilia) inherited as an autosomal dominant trait with variable expression (factor VIII deficiency). Careful examination of affected and related animals is undertaken by certain vets to identify the problem. Treatment is most easily accomplished by transfusion of fresh compatible plasma at regular intervals once any acquired clotting defects have been eliminated.

Insurance

An increasing number of owners are realising the value of pet insurance. Third party and veterinary fees are included in many 'packages'. Preventive medicine is not covered but the insurance companies do recognise the value of such measures. A variety of schemes are available – some payments are made direct to the practice – all of which encourage the fullest veterinary care following injury or disease. Visit your practice and discuss the policies available there.

Kidney, hepatic and cardiac disease

Very briefly, I would like to consider three inter-related groups of problems.

KIDNEY DISEASE

Infection, poisoning and hypertension can lead to renal failure. Some infectious forms have already been mentioned. General wear and tear due mostly to age (nephrosis) is to be expected. A slight increase in thirst flushes the kidneys to compensate for inefficient filtration but more protein than normal is lost in the urine so often a weight loss is noticed. When protein loss is severe, general oedema (fluid under skin and a distended abdomen) is seen. A high protein, low salt and a potassium-enriched diet (fruit) should be given. Inability to concentrate urine and excessive thirst and urination may also involve the kidneys. This requires careful investigation by your vet to ascertain the possible cause(s). Oedema leads to the next general group of problems – cardiac and hepatic disease.

HEPATIC DISEASE

Viruses, bacteria and certain worm larvae (ascarids) invade the liver causing disruption of function and cells. Scarring (cirrhosis) and bile flow obstruction (jaundice) can result as well as the reduced ability to synthesize protein (causing oedema.) Diseases such as diabetes mellitus or canine Cushing's Disease (hyperactivity of the adrenal glands) will elevate blood sugar levels and cause an enlargement of the liver.

CARDIAC DISEASE

This may be a result of developing defects of the heart valves and blood vessels, arising from wear and tear, infection (bacterial infection of valves, parvo-virus infection of muscle cells), occasionally heart blood vessel circulation failure (heart attack), or with congenital defects and tumours.

Leaky valves create sounds made recognisable by using the stethoscope which can also identify excessively irregular rapid or slow heart beats. Congestive heart failure can start with such problems. A sluggish blood flow through the lungs accumulates excess fluid which shows up as a heart cough (especially at night), laboured breathing and exercise intolerance, poor collection of blood from the abdomen (ascites ballooned out) and enlarged liver.

Routine checkups are advised by most vets often after every 2 to 3 heart tablet prescriptions simply to ensure that the dose/drug is still effective or necessary and to take the opportunity for a general health check up.

Regular exercise and attention to diet (keeping to a suitable weight especially if spayed or castrated) is important (as I refer to in the obesity section) both to help prevent the condition from developing or relapsing from a compensated state. Low salt, adequate roughage and protein diets are advised. Enzyme injections and diuretics are used in canine heart disease as in human cases.

Mental problems

Some of the mental problems which may be recognised in individual dogs can involve separation anxiety (also fear of solitude) boredom (leading to self-mutilation), depraved appetite, fear of the car, motion or thunder and overactivity leading to hysteria.

Homoeopathy plus attention to the diet (with or without conventional medicine) generally has good effect.

Neuroses

Highly-strung dogs, dogs which are simply neurotic or those dogs such as the Dobermann which need a lot of exercise and are not getting enough, may develop skin diseases by continually licking themselves. They usually find a spot and just keep licking themselves until the hair gets licked away, the skin thickens and then breaks to ooze serum or whole blood. The whole process could take from one to several days and is worth early detection to avoid discomfort and blemishing.

TREATMENT

Apply calamine lotion to affected spot.
If the dog continues to chew and lick it may be necessary to bandage the area.

Put on an Elizabethan collar.

Try and make sure the dog is exercised properly to use up the excess energy and give him something to look forward to each day.

Consult your veterinary surgeon, before wet eczema and a 'lick granuloma' develops.

Nursing elderly dogs

Old dogs present special problems and their general condition can be greatly improved simply by feeding them good quality food in proper amounts.

When nursing older dogs whose appetite might not be all it should, encourage appetite by feeding meat extracts and flavourings. Since a dog's sense of smell and taste fades with age, some extra attention to an appetising diet will be necessary to keep him interested in food.

Some elderly dogs suffer from kidney problems. If this is the case, they should be fed a low protein diet composed of white meat (rabbit, fish, or chicken) with rice or biscuit meal mixed in. Supplement the diet with good quality vitamin and mineral additives.

Elderly dogs should be given all the water they require and make sure the water bowl is always full. See Chapter on Feeding the Older Dog.

Nursing a sick dog

If your dog is suffering from a severe or debilitating disease and is too weak and sick to feed itself, the nursing and loving care you give your friend will have a vital effect on recovery to good health.

1 Keep sick dogs in a warm, quiet and dimly lit room, and try not to disturb them too often.

2 Keep him clean and special care should be taken if he is suffering from diarrhoea or vomiting. All animals are fastidious and become quite upset if allowed to foul themselves. If this has happened then they should be gently washed with soap and water.

3 If a dog is so weak and unable to move himself then he should be turned regularly every four hours to prevent bed sores.

4 A sick dog is best left alone as much as possible apart from doing what is necessary for its well being. Never fuss the dog – there is a difference between loving care and fussing.

DIET FOR A SICK DOG

Sick dogs and dogs recuperating from an illness need very nourishing food and may need to be coaxed to eat, because they won't feel like eating. Supplement their diet with a mixture of four tablespoons glucose to one pint of water daily, this gives them extra energy. However do not give this or any rich fluids to a dog that is vomiting – 1 rounded dessertspoon/pint water given 10–15 mls three times hourly. The dog may feel hungry but do not feed him all at one time. It is far better to feed little and often at regular intervals. If the dog has no appetite, try to tempt him with foods such as chicken, cheese, fish, salmon, tinned sardines. Home-made meat extracts often do the trick and are made by mincing meat as finely as possible and then pouring boiling water over the minced meat. The liquid is then poured into a bowl with a pinch of salt.

Make every effort to tempt the dog to eat voluntarily. Forced-feeding is a last resort. Remember the smallest amount of food taken voluntarily and regularly will do more in the long run than a large amount forced down.

HYGIENE

All utensils which come in contact with the dog must be sterilised in boiling water or hypochlorite after each meal. Scrupulous hygiene is essential to successful nursing.

Obesity

This is becoming more widely recognised as a controllable problem. There are marked differences in obesity between breeds but, within each breed, older dogs have a lower metabolic rate and are less active. Bitches are more likely to be obese than males with neutering decreasing activity further in both sexes.

Obesity can exacerbate certain pre-existing skeletal and joint diseases as well as creating circulatory problems. The latter may lead to increased risk during anaesthesia and surgical procedures which is not helped by the deposition of fat in the liver cells.

When obesity is not caused by any endocrine hormone disease, regular weighing, palpation and observation can lead to early recognition of the problem.

Calorie restriction intake with better exercise may be achieved at home with or without proprietary low calorie diets. During the weight reduction period, weekly or fortnightly checks on the dog's weight should be made and a maintenance diet adhered to when a satisfactory weight reduction is achieved.

The oestrus cycle and spaying

The reproductive cycle of the bitch is divided into sections – that leading up to heat, the actual heat itself then the waning phase after the true heat. Swelling of the vulva with visible blood is usually followed by standing to the dog around 13 days later (true oestrus phase). The resting reproductive state is normally reached some three months after oestrus and this is the stage when spaying (should it be required) is best undertaken with the least tissue loss to the bitch.

It is unwise to spay a pseudo-pregnant bitch even at this time since the condition can be intensified as well as additional tissue trauma from the usually enlarged, engorged udder. Antiprolactin drugs may be used to correct the hormonal inbalance before spaying.

Pregnancy diagnosis

May be undertaken at 2 to 3 weeks after mating. Where only one pup is present it may be 'lost' into the part of the abdomen covered by the ribs when a late presentation is made. Your vet may wish to re-examine in a further week or two when other signs of pregnancy may be more pronounced.

Calcification of the puppy's skeleton occurs at the 5 to 6 weeks stage (the skeleton would now show up on radiographs). When the bitch is taken to the vet this is a good opportunity to make sure that the nutritional supplements and diet will be adequate throughout the pre-and-post whelping stages. Your visit will also act as a mental note for your vet as to when the whelping will be due.

Skin

GENERAL CARE

The skin is a very important organ which acts as an indicator for internal body problems but it may act as the *only* indicator and is the barrier between internal organs of the body and the environment. Thus it indicates injuries, hormonal disease, systemic infections, diet, metabolic disease (liver dysfunction), parasitism and allergy.

DANDRUFF

Is a common problem. It can reflect internal problems such as reduced thyroid activity when associated with hair loss on head and
body and lethargy. It can be helped by additional, balanced coat
conditioning powder or liquids, by biotin (Vit.H) or by conditioning,
tar/sulphur, or chlorhexidine shampoos. It can also arise from im-
proper rinsing of unsuitable shampoos. Regular grooming with shampoos only when necessary will aid skin care and make an opportunity
for regular examination for health.

PARASITES AND THE SKIN

Young pups are often parasitised by grey/brown-coloured lice (egg
cases may be seen attached to hairs) and mahogany coloured fleas.
Nit combs and flea combs usually demonstrate the problem. Fleas
may be present at any stage of the dog's life and have both environmental and host parts to their life cycle. Even after a year or more, in
an empty house fleas, emerge from egg cases when stimulated by
vibrations, carbon dioxide and warmth. When a flea is seen passing
over the head hair or suspicious bites appear on an owner's ankles
and arms then a flea comb plus insecticidal spray/powder should be
used and the bedding changed. When dogs are left to become seething
flea circuses, repetitive hoovering and environmental flea control is
very necessary. These dogs often show hair loss and eczema from
allergic reaction to the flea saliva.

Mange mites can also be present. Demodectic mange may not be
a clinical problem if the dog's skin and the mite are in neutrality
(living together in harmony). However, if the mite population ex-
plodes and spreads from the vibrissae and small whiskers and eyelids
into the chin and body skin follicles, then severe reactions can occur,
often with pus in the follicles. In my opinion this is the main cause
of chin spots.

Not as common is the mange mite *Sarcoptes* which often is seen to
cause limb skin inflammation and hair loss. These mites are much
more active and capable of transmission to other dogs.

A walk on sunny common land or sheep grazing often collect the
odd tick: these start off small, dark, black/grey rice grain-sized and,
after feeding, enlarge to a pale grey/cream cherry-stone size. It is not
always easy to see the small ticks but large ticks can be removed by
careful anti-clockwise unscrewing (untwist the mouth parts which, if
left in, cause a marked reaction), by neat Dettol, a lighted cigarette-
end to the free end or in the last resort an insecticidal spray.

Stings

Often occur on eyelids, nose, ears or neck. A wasp's sting is best treated by cold compress of neat vinegar (except near eye). A bee sting is left behind usually and should be removed as soon as possible. Then a cold, strong bicarbonate compress can be applied (except near the eye). This action can be followed by antihistamine cream. Severe reactions and multiple stings should be seen professionally *as soon as possible* after they have occurred.

Ant stings seem to cause the most marked swelling of a dog's muzzle and these cases should be given antihistamine by mouth and by injection as soon as possible to prevent eye and throat complications.

Taking a dog's temperature

This is not difficult and the technique is quite simple. The type of thermometer to be used is any stubby-bulbed *clinical* thermometer and are available at all chemists or from your vet. The technique for taking a dog's temperature must always be taken via the rectum *never by mouth*.

Have someone hold the dog, a well trained animal should not make too much fuss. Shake thermometer down to 95°F (35°C) and it is best to do this while standing the dog over a rug or towel, just in case you happen to drop the thermometer it won't shatter. Dip the bulb of the thermometer in Vaseline. Approach the dog from the rear and gently slide an inch of the thermometer through the anal sphincter. Be prepared to stop the dog from sitting down. Once the thermometer is in place support protruding end and wait one minute. Withdraw thermometer and wipe it with a Kleenex or cottonwool and read the temperature carefully.

Normal body temperature (average) for a dog is 101·3°F (38·5°C) (N.B. range – 100·9°F – 101·7°F) 38·3–38·7°C. A temperature of 102·5°F (39·2°C) and higher is significant and a good reason to consult your vet.

When finished with the thermometer wash it in *cold* water and dip it in alcohol before wiping and putting away. Always keep this thermometer strictly for your dog's use only.

Taking samples of faeces and urine

As dogs never 'perform' at the most convenient time when you want them to and most certainly never when you are watching them you too have to be crafty and make out you really do not want anything from them. The best time to collect a sample is first thing in the morning. Collect the sample of faeces immediately and put in a tin or plastic container with a lid on, clearly labelled with the dog's name, owner's name and address and the date.

Collecting a urine sample is more difficult. One way is to use a sheet of polythene with a dent shape in the centre – let the dog sniff it first and he will hopefully urinate over it and the dent in the centre will hopefully collect a pool. Transfer to a clean bottle or jar.

With a bitch it might be better to watch her carefully and, just as she is about to sit down, stick a saucer underneath her, or a plastic tray on a long handle. Only a few mls. are necessary for laboratory analysis.

Techniques of administering tablets and pills

Try concealing the pill in a tasty titbit – cheese or a piece of meat. Some dogs are notorious at finding the most cunningly concealed pill – if you cannot conceal the pill in something tasty, then I am afraid it is the 'no messing about' technique i.e. the direct approach.

Open the dog's mouth and place the tablet down the throat as far as possible. Hold the jaw shut and stroke the throat. Make a fuss of it afterwards.

Travelling

Sedation with specially timed acetylpromazine or primidone medication rarely works without making the dog unreasonably sleepy long after arrival from the journey. I have suggested junior travel sickness tablets and also passed on advice on how to accustom the young and growing dog to the car. Travel sickness can be present as excess salivation with an apprehensive or depressed expression, possibly with vomiting.

Homoeopathic remedies such as widely curative Petroleum may be used with also Borax, Cocculus and Tabacum to consider. Hyoscyamus could be considered in cases of excessive in-car excitement.

Veterinary homoeopathy

I would now like to lead into veterinary homoeopathy in a little more detail.

An increasing number of vets are becoming aware of the opportunities offered by homoeopathic material in successfully helping the body to heal itself rapidly and completely. In many cases, especially good results are achieved with conventional veterinary medicine or where a combination of the two ways of treatment is made. After thorough clinical examination of the patient, homoeopathy involves the careful selection of a substance suitable to cure a disease by the knowledge that this same substance 'in the raw' could cause the same signs as seen in the patient.

An integral part of homoeopathy is the principle of the minimal dose – the potentised remedy is given in sufficient dose to overcome the disease without the need to worry about the potential toxicity associated with the 'raw' material. The raw substance is diluted stage by stage and agitated at each stage in order to release the purified curative energy of the substance whilst the dilution removes any toxic and harmful effects. Homoeopathic remedies can therefore be used in the knowledge that even if the wrong remedy is chosen, while it will achieve no cure, it will do no harm.

There are therefore no side effects, no suppression of signs which reappear later (perhaps worse, like itchy skins). A careful evaluation of the signs and symptoms enables one to treat animals with both diagnosed and undiagnosed disease. It involves whole patient treatment when the chosen substance works with the body's own defence mechanisms to effect a cure. Homoeopathy is worth serious consideration.

Vital Facts and Figures

Respiration Rate: 15 to 30 breaths per minute at rest.
Pulse Rate: 70–100 per minute at rest.
Rectal Temperature: Between 100·9 and 101·7°F (38·3 and 38·7°C) mostly 101·3 or 38·5°C.
Body Weight of Adult – male – 80–85 lb (36·4–38·6 kg)
                             – female – 70–75 lb (31·8–34·1 kg)

Worms

These are important internal parasites of both young and mature animals. The roundworm infestation of pups takes place via the placenta and via the milk after birth. It is to be expected that only very stringent worming of the bitch will prevent puppy infection due to such a life cycle. Pups may start being wormed at monthly intervals starting from four weeks of age up to six months then twice yearly.

A pot-bellied, unthrifty puppy with occasional vomiting or diarrhoea and a poor, scurfy, staring coat generally carries worms. In the vomit or diarrhoea worms may be present with their eggs. The worms are between 2″ and 6″ (50 and 150mm) long and an offwhite/beige colour, straight, curved or coiled up. There have been reported instances of the roundworm larvae present in these eggs hatching after inadvertent ingestion by children to cause eye disease. Such a zoonosis (disease transmissible from animal to human) must demand preventative measures.

Tapeworm infection is most common in mature animals and often involves fleas since these external parasites carry immature tapeworms inside their bodies. During grooming, the flea is eaten and so the life cycle is completed. Certain immature tapeworms are present in the head and abdomen of dead sheep perhaps found not buried on hillsides or after snowdrifts have thawed. Offal from such carcases will pass on the tape worms into the dog which will spread them onto pasture from its faeces (and also to us as it is a zoonosis). This is why farm dogs are wormed regularly. Rarely a dog may catch and eat a rabbit or other wild animal and so collect another tapeworm. It is wise to worm older dogs with combined round tapewormers at least twice yearly and also to control any fleas.

12   First Aid

In this chapter I have included some rudimentary advice on first aid but I cannot stress too strongly the importance of consulting your vet if you are in any doubts.

Animal bites

SIGNS

Punctures or tears in the skin. Hair matted with blood. Licking bitten parts. Swelling.

ACTION

Clip hair around wound with blunt tipped scissors. Flush wound with three per cent solution of hydrogen peroxide. Wash thoroughly with germicidal soap and water. Thoroughly rinse all soap away and any lingering hairs with a jet of water from a squeezable, clean plastic bottle.

Apply antiseptic cream to a superficial wound and check regularly for signs of infection, followed by a wound powder once the wound has stopped discharging. If the wound is deep after cleaning it, or if there is a skin flap, arrange to see your veterinary surgeon as soon as possible – large wounds often can be sutured when they are fresh.

Artificial respiration

Artificial respiration does the work of normal breathing, pushing air into and out of the dog's lungs. It should be administered as soon as it is seen that the animal is not breathing. Delay in acting can be fatal. Within two or three minutes after breathing stops, the dog may be beyond recovery.

ACTION:

1 Lay the dog on its right side.
2 Open the dog's mouth and check that there are no obstructions to breathing. If there are any obstructions (e.g. stones, gravel, sand, socks, tights) pull them out with your fingers. Make sure that the tongue is lolling out and clear of the back of the throat.
3 Place the flat of both hands below the shoulder blade and over the ribs.
4 Press down firmly to empty the lungs.
5 Release the pressure. The lungs should fill as the natural elasticity of the chest returns to its normal position.
6 Repeat pressing down and releasing the pressure every five seconds until the dog is breathing on its own again. This could take up to an hour.
7 The movements should be brisk and forceful. Press down hard. Release suddenly.

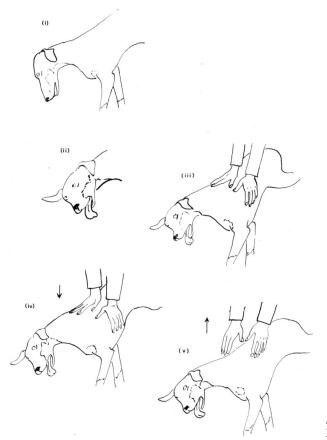

Artificial
Respiration.

MOUTH TO MOUTH RESUSCITATION

It is simple enough. Just hold the dog's mouth closed and blow into its nostrils. Wait a second and blow again. The idea is to inflate the animal's lungs with air so that they function of their own accord.

ARTIFICIAL RESPIRATION – SWINGING TECHNIQUE (Puppies and small dogs)

1   Slap the dog sharply on the side once or twice.
2   Lift the dog by its hind legs, extend your arms and swing it back and forth ten times. Wait a few seconds for a gasp and if there is none swing the animal again.
3   When you swing a dog this way, the weight of the abdominal contents will contract and expand the lungs. If after four such swinging sessions the dog is still not breathing then administer mouth to mouth resuscitation (see illustration).

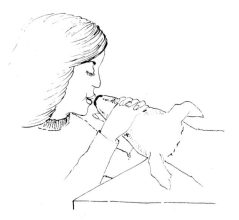

Mouth to Mouth
Resuscitation.

Bleeding

SIGNS

From artery, bright red blood gushes from injury. From vein, dark red blood flows steadily from injury. (Often mixed together). From capillaries, blood can seep or ooze at a slower rate, often in beads from the wound surface.

ACTION

Control bleeding with pressure bandage. Apply gauze dressing, clean handkerchief or clean napkin over wound and apply pressure with fingers or palms of hands. Cold compresses can shut down surface bleeding. If bleeding does not stop add more packing on top of original dressing and continue pressure. Get someone to ring your vet to arrange admission and be prepared to use a tourniquet on heart side of the wound if blood loss is threatening life. Then get to your vet, as soon as possible.

Car accident

SIGNS

In pain. Concussed. Possibly parts of body (especially legs and back) paralysed. Leg hanging and unable to support dog's weight. Limping.

ACTION

Beware of being bitten. Do not move dog unless absolutely necessary, until you determine the extent of injuries.
1   See that dog can breathe freely.
2   Stop bleeding with a pressure bandage. Use gauze or a clean hankie and apply pressure with fingers over wound.
3   Ask someone to ring your vet to arrange admission.
4   Support broken bones with newspapers, towels, cotton wool and bandages if possible.
5   Keep dog warm and quiet.
6   Move dog carefully if injuries are serious, remembering any extra advice your vet may have given you. Using a blanket as a stretcher put the dog straight into the car or if spinal injuries are suspected first onto a small door, then the car. Keep outwardly calm and be reassuring to your dog for as long as you can.

Choking

SIGNS

Gulping. Gagging. Gasping for breath. Excessive salivation. Pawing at mouth. Dog very distressed.

ACTION

Open mouth and try to retrieve object with your fingers or pliers. If you cannot lay dog on its side place palms of your hands on dog's rib cage and press down sharply to expel the foreign body from throat. Open mouth to locate and remove object.

Diarrhoea

SIGNS

Loose bowel motions. Persistent wet, soft, cowpat version of normal, colour ranging through to abnormal bright yellowy/pink/red/black and foetid smelling. Blood may be seen even when of normal colour.

ACTION

Stop all food for 18 to 24 hours. Using water which has been boiled and with one rounded dessert spoon glucose added per pint, allow small regular amounts to be drunk throughout the day. This will prevent dehydration. Kaolin and morphine could also be given. However, if vomiting is present the latter mixture would be too strong for a sensitive stomach and fluids given would have to be one or two teaspoons only three or four times an hour. By now, with diarrhoea and vomiting you should be taking your dog to a vet. With diarrhoea only, once the dog has been starved for 24 hours try very small light meals – cottage cheese, scrambled eggs, boiled rice and potatoes. Should such diarrhoea last for 24 to 36 hours consult your vet but do so earlier especially if your dog is showing noticeable distress in attempting to pass diarrhoea.

Electric shock

SIGNS

Pale bluish and cold skin. Low temperature, irregular heartbeat, burns on lip and tongue, collapse, respiratory failure.

ACTION

If cord is still in contact with any part of the dog's body use a broom handle or some other non-conductor of electricity to push it away. Listen to the dog's chest by placing your ear behind its elbow to find out about the heart beat. If you hear nothing or if it is very fast and faint (plus a blue tongue) then immediately, rapidly, and repetitively compress the heart area using the palms of your hands to establish a heart beat. Keep your dog warm and quiet. Possibly offer a drink of sugared tea if it is thirsty and get the dog to the vet immediately.

Eye problems

SIGNS

Depend on injury but the dog scratching its eyes, excessive blinking and tear formation are signs. Also cut or bleeding eyelids and blood-shot eyes.

ACTION

Eyes are very delicate and easily injured. Except for small foreign bodies that you can dislodge by flushing the eyes with warm water or carefully lifting out with a moistened cotton wool swab and soap or chemical irritations, when the eyes should be flushed immediately with warm water, all other injuries should be handled by a vet.

Foot problems

SIGNS

Limping. Chewing toes or footpads. Bleeding. Swelling and redness.

ACTION

Remove foreign objects with cotton swabs or tweezers. Large chunks of glass or nails deeply embedded should be removed by a vet. Stop bleeding, wash area with germicidal soap and water. Flush wound with 3 per cent hydrogen peroxide. Apply antiseptic. Bandage to prevent infection. Have deep wounds treated by vet.

Frostbite

SIGNS

Cold, bluish or pale skin.

ACTION

Handle dog gently. Rewarm skin slowly with moist heat; tepid water bottle or repetitive tepid water compresses. While warming do not massage affected areas to increase circulation. See vet immediately in extreme cases.

Gastric torsion

SIGNS

Sudden death. Extreme shock, swollen abdomen. Cold extremities.

PREVENTION

Soak complete foods thoroughly. Do not allow access to source of dry food and feed only to age and weight and not to appetite.

ACTION

If not too far advanced, this is an extreme emergency requiring gastric decompression and sometimes surgical correction by your vet.

Heat stroke

Most often caused when a dog is locked in a car or travel cage without air in hot weather. If a car has a sun roof always leave it open in hot weather plus two inches of the door windows all round to get an air current.

SIGNS

Heavy panting. Dazed expression. Gasping for breath. Muscle twitching. Staggering gait. High temperature. Convulsions and collapse.

ACTION

Move dog to a cool place. Wet it all over with cool water to remove heat from body preferably soaking the whole body in a sink, bath or in a tub and sluicing cold water over dog's back. The tongue colour can change from mottled blue/red to a healthier pink. If no thermometer is available, once tongue pinkens and a comfortable breathing rate is established, water cooling can stop and then dab the dripping fur dry. Ice-packs could be used through a handkerchief if running water is not available but this will take longer. If, despite first aid, coughing with foamy saliva, laboured breathing, a poor tongue colour still remains or gets worse, see the vet immediately.

Obnoxious odours

SIGNS

Unpleasant smell. Possibly also infected anal glands.

ACTION

Bath dog with coal tar/baby shampoo or wheatgerm/conditioning shampoo to remove dirt and debris. Rinse well. Towel dry. Use solution of a proprietary brand odour remover. Follow with canine cologne to mask any remaining odours.

Poison inhaled

SIGNS

Nausea and dizziness. Respiratory problems. Staggering gait. Loss of consciousness. Convulsions.

ACTION

Remove dog from toxic environment to fresh air. Get to vet at once for oxygen and medical treatment, provide him with information on nature of poison.

Poison skin contact

From sitting, rolling or walking on toxic surfaces or from poisonous substances on coat and skin.

SIGNS

Skin reactions depends on substance and include redness, rash, skin peeling.

ACTION

Flush skin with luke warm water to remove unabsorbed materials. Then, if substance contained an acid, rinse skin with a mixture of three tablespoons baking soda dissolved in 1 quart of warm water. If it contained an alkali, rinse with equal parts of vinegar and water or, if it contained paint thinners, solvents or gasoline for example, saturate skin with milk or vegetable oil. Shampoo fifteen minutes later. For tar or oil, use a gel hand-cleanser and then wash off.

Poison swallowed

SIGNS

They depend on toxic substance but include trembling, shivering, dilated pupils, vomiting, diarrhoea, staggering gait, increased salivation, convulsions (sometimes) coma.

ACTION

If antidote appears on package label of product ingested, follow directions. If not, call vet immediately and give as much information as possible about what dog swallowed. Depending on poison you will either (1) induce vomiting to remove unabsorbed portion from dog's body using two large washing soda crystals or (2) if poison cannot be vomited, dilute and delay further absorption by giving milk, whipped egg whites, vegetable or mineral oil or water. Get dog to the vet immediately.

Seizure

SIGNS

Excessive salivation. Muscle twitching. Wide-eyed expression. Involuntary movement.

ACTION

Do not restrain. Do not put any type of medication into dog's mouth. Keep children away. Cover with towel or blanket to keep warm. When seizure subsides, keep dog quiet and warm. If seizures are prolonged or recurrent see your vet. Refer to detailed paragraphs in veterinary section.

Vomiting

SIGNS

Restlessness. Increased salivation, licking lips and frequent swallowing. Intermittent abdominal contractions.

ACTION

Stop all food for 12 to 24 hours. If dog is thirsty, give very small regular amounts of cooled boiled water or soda water. When vomiting stops feed bland food, nothing fatty. Consult your vet. Refer to detailed paragraphs in veterinary section.

First Aid cupboard

This should only include a few essentials for minor incidents.

Poisoning and bad sting reactions should be treated by your vet. In cases of suspected poisoning it is helpful to take a sample of whatever is thought to have caused it to your vet. Stings may need antihistamine treatment. This is why amateur first aid is not recommended on these apart from removing the sting if possible. Remember, vinegar for wasp stings and bicarbonate of soda for bee stings.

Ice cubes should be kept for emergencies and used as an icepack should throat or mouth be affected.

An animal thermometer is essential but do not be fooled that if a dog isn't running a temperature he is not ill. If he looks off colour, more than likely he is.

You need an efficient pair of tweezers and eyebrow forceps are useful for removing deeply embedded thorns and other foreign bodies including grass seeds. (Grass seeds with hooks under third eyelid must not be messed about with, that's a vet's job.) You will also need:
Blunt-ended scissors: for cutting plasters and bandages and trimming hair around the wounds.
Rolls of bandages and cotton wool.
Roll of elastoplast.
Sterile dressings (unopened). (Never fasten bandages with pins or safety pins).
A knob of bitter aloes on bandage (sticky when wet) discourages animal from chewing bandage.
Washing soda (makes dog sick when it has swallowed Warfarin, gloves, tights etc).
Antiseptic in tube.
Friars Balsam applied neat to pink sweating foot sores.
Bottle of kaolin and morphine mixture from vet for mild cases of diarrhoea.
Liquid paraffin.
Epsom salts to bathe scratches.
Tubes of ointment (which must be fresh so infection is not passed on).
Glucose to make up as a drink for sick dogs.
Benylin for coughs.
Dettol, TCP or liquid Savlon.
Coopers louse powder for defleaing.

List of poisons found in the house, garage and garden

Aspirin, paracetamol etc.
Sleeping tablets
Tranquillisers
Mothballs
Bleach
Lavatory cleaners
Dry cleaning fluids
Laundry blue
Nappy washes
Soap powders
Upholstery cleaners
Drain cleaners
Matches
Oven cleaners
Tobacco, cigars
Spoiled food
Antiseptics
Antifreeze
Brake fluids
Petrol
Kerosene
Motor oil
Insecticide sprays
Paints and thinners
Weed killers
Slug and snail baits
Rat, mouse, ant and cockroach poisons
Paraquat
Fungicides
Sheep and cattle dips

Appendix 1

Useful addresses

Central Dog Registry (Mrs A. Stone)   49 Marloes Road, London W8 6LA. 01 572-7848

Dobermann Rescue Ltd   61 Park Mead, Sidcup, Kent. 01 304-2942

Dog Breeders Associates Co   1 Abbey Road, Bourne End, Bucks. SL8 5N2. Bourne End 20943/29000

Dog Breeders Insurance Co Ltd   12 Christchurch Road, Lansdowne, Bournemouth BH1 3LE. Bournemouth 295771

Dogs Monthly   Unit 1, Bowen Industrial Estate, Aberbargoed, Bargoed, Mid Glamorgan CF8 9ET

Dog World   The Churchyard, Ashford, Kent. *Ashford* 21877

The Kennel Club   1 Clarges Street, London W1. 01 493-6651

National Boarding Kennels Association   c/o Blue Grass Animal Hotel, Little Leigh, Northwich, Cheshire.

National Canine Defence   1 and 2 Pratt Mews, London NW1 0AD. 01 388-0137

Our Dogs   Oxford Road, Station Approach, Manchester M60 1SX. 061-236-2660

Pet Crematoria   Our Dogs, Oxford Road, Station Approach, Manchester M60 1SX

Pet Plan Ltd   319–327 Chiswick High Road, London W4 4HH

Private Pet Policies (*Vetwise, & Vetex*)   Orient House, 42–45 New Broadstreet, London EC2 M1QY. 01 628-0305

PRO Dogs National Charity   Rocky Bank, 4 New Road, Ditton, Maidstone, Kent. 0732-848499

R.S.P.C.A.   The Causeway, Horsham, Sussex

Appendix 2

1. Foreface

2. Stop

3. Forehead

4. Neck

5. Withers

6. Back

7. Croup

8. Loin

9. Thigh

10. Hock joint

11. Hock

12. Second Thigh

13. Stifle

14. Tuck-up

15. Brisket

16. Ribs

17. Shoulders

18. Pastern

19. Elbow

20. Fore chest

21. Neck

22. Cheek

23. Flews

24. Chin

The Dobermann Breed Standard

CHARACTERISTICS

The Dobermann is a dog of good medium size with a well set body, muscular and elegant. He has a proud carriage and a bold, alert temperament. His form is compact and tough and owing to his build capable of great speed. His gait is light and elastic. His eyes show intelligence and firmness of character, and he is loyal and obedient. Shyness or viciousness must be heavily penalised.

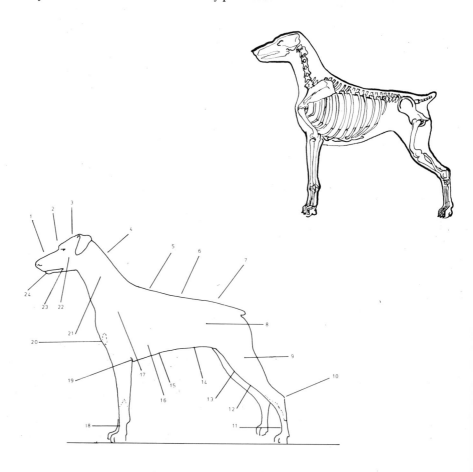

HEAD AND SKULL

Has to be proportionate to the body. It must be long, well filled under the eyes and clean cut. Its form seen from above and from the side must resemble a blunt wedge. The upper part of the head should be as flat as possible and free from wrinkle. The top of the skull should be flat with a slight stop, and the muzzle line extend parallel to the top line of the skull. The cheeks must be flat and the lips tight. The nose should be solid black in black dogs, solid dark brown in brown dogs and solid grey in blue dogs. Head out of balance in proportion to body, dish-faced, snipey or cheeky should be penalised.

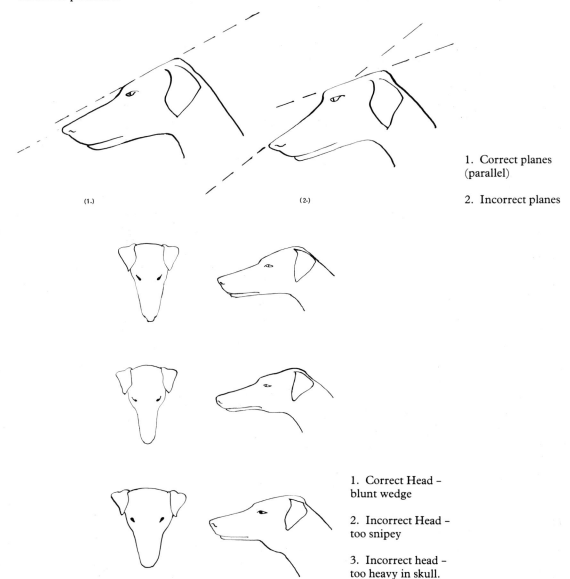

(1.)   (2.)

1. Correct planes (parallel)

2. Incorrect planes

1. Correct Head – blunt wedge

2. Incorrect Head – too snipey

3. Incorrect head – too heavy in skull.

EYES

Should be almond shaped, not round, moderately deep set, not prominent, with vigorous, energetic expression. Iris of uniform colour, ranging from medium to darkest brown in black dogs, the darker shade being the more desirable. In browns or blues the colour of the iris should blend with that of the markings, but not to be of lighter hue than that of the markings. Light eyes in black dogs to be discouraged.

EARS

Should be small, neat and set high on the head. Erect or dropped, but erect preferred.

MOUTH

Should be very well developed, solid and strong, with a scissor bite. The incisors of the lower jaw must touch the inner face of the incisors of the upper jaw. Overshot or undershot mouths, badly arranged or decayed teeth to be penalised.

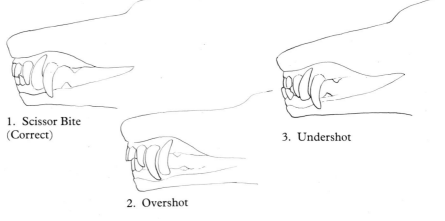

1. Scissor Bite
(Correct)

2. Overshot

3. Undershot

NECK

Should be fairly long and lean, carried erect and with considerable nobility, slightly convex and proportionate to the whole shape of the dog. The region of the nape has to be muscular. Dewlap and loose skin are undesirable.

FOREQUARTERS

The shoulder blade and upper arm should meet at an angle of 90°. Relative length of shoulder and upper arm should be as one, excess length of upper arm being much less undesirable than excess length of shoulder blade. The legs, seen from the front and side, are perfectly straight and parallel to each other from elbow to pastern, muscled and sinewy, with round bone proportionate to body structure. In a normal position and when gaiting the elbow should lie close to the brisket.

BODY

Should be square, height measured vertically from the ground to the highest point of the withers, equalling the length measured horizontally, from the forechest to rear projection of the upper thigh. The back should be short and firm with the topline sloping slightly from the withers to the croup, the female needing more room to carry litters may be slightly longer to loin. The belly should be fairly well tucked up. Ribs should be deep and well-sprung reaching to elbow. Long, weak or roach backs to be discouraged.

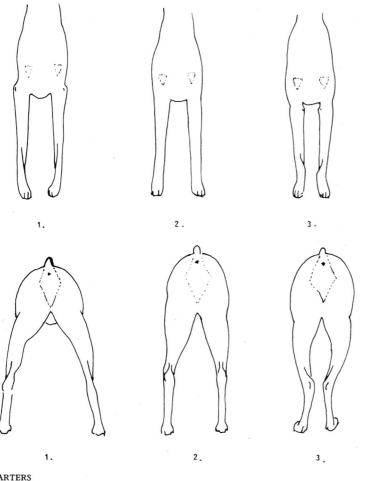

1. Elbows out

2. Normal front

3. Cabriole front

1. Too wide hindquarters

2. Correct hindquarters

3. Cow hocks

HINDQUARTERS

Should be parallel to each other and wide enough apart to fit in with a properly built body. The hip bone should fall away from the spinal column at an angle of about 30°. Croup well filled out. The hindquarters should be well developed and muscular, with long bent stifle and their hocks turning neither in nor out. While the dog is at rest, hock to heel should be perpendicular to the ground.

FEET

Forefeet should be well arched, compact and cat like, turning neither in nor out. All dew claws should be removed. Long, flat, deviating paws and weak pasterns should be penalised. Hind feet should be well arched, compact and cat like, turning neither in nor out.

GAIT

Should be free, balanced and vigorous with good reach in the forequarters and a driving power in the hind quarters. When trotting there should be a strong rear action drive with rotary motion of the hind quarters. Rear and front legs should be thrown neither in nor out. Back should remain strong and firm.

TAIL

The tail should be docked at the first or second joint and should appear to be a continuation of the spine, without material drop.

COAT

Should be smooth haired, short, hard and thick and close lying. Invisible grey under-coat on neck permissible.

COLOUR

Colours allowed are definite black, brown, blue or isabella (fawn) with rust red markings. Markings must be sharply defined and appearing above each eye and on the muzzle, throat and forechest, and on all legs and feet and below tail. White markings of any kind are highly undesirable.

WEIGHT AND SIZE

Ideal height at withers: Males 27 inches, Females 25½ inches. Considerable deviation from this ideal to be discouraged.

FAULTS

Shyness or viciousness must be heavily penalised.
Head out of balance in proportion to body, dish-faced, snipey or cheeky should be penalised.
Light eyes in black dogs should be discouraged.
Dewlap and loose skin are undesirable.
Overshot or undershot mouths, badly arranged or decayed teeth to be penalised.
Long, weak or roach backs to be discouraged.
White markings of any kind are highly undesirable.
Hair forming a ridge on the back of the neck and/or along the spine should be classed as a serious fault.

Reprinted with the kind permission of The Kennel Club.

Appendix 3

Glossary of terms

Allergy   Specific or *morgeneral hypersensitivity*.

Alopecia   Loss of hair.

Anaemia   Generally a deficiency of red blood cells. A common cause is severe infestation of parasites.

Anal glands   The two glands situated slightly below and to the side of the anus. Sometimes become blocked and need to be emptied.

Anthelmintics   A drug which kills parasitic worms and sometimes their eggs and larvae.

Arthritis   Inflammation of the joints. Deep heat and rest are essential and important, as this can be a very painful condition.

Ascarids   Type of roundworm.

Ascites   Fluid in the abdomen.

Ataxia   Loss of control of movements.

Balanitis   Inflammation of the dog's sheath, which may include the penis (*balanoposthitis*).

Benched show   A dog show where all dogs are benched on benches and secured to the bench by a collar and benching chain.

Benching chain   Collar and chain used to secure dog on bench.

Biopsy   Small portion of living tissue which is examined as an aid to diagnosis.

Black tripe   Food for dog. Can be bought either direct from abattoirs or minced and packed from petshops or animal food farms.

Blue   Dark grey.

Breed standard   The official description of the breed to which dogs should be judged.

Canine Cushings Disease   Occurs in a dog usually after five years of age. Caused by excessive production of cortico steroids by the adrenal cortex.

Canine parvo virus   An infectious virus extremely serious and contagious. Vaccination absolutely essential and reinforced with boosters annually.

Cervical spondylolithesis (also cervical vertebral instability – C.V.I.)   'Wobbler' syndrome, narrowing of the spinal canal and variable compression of spinal cord from deformed and displaced neck vertebrae.

Character   The make-up of the dog combining all essential points of appearance, disposition and behaviour.

Choke collar   A chain or leather or nylon collar that loosens or tightens according to what is required by the handler.

Cleft palate   A congenital defect in which two bony halves of the hard palate fail to unite along centre line leaving a gap between them.

Colostrum   A secretion of the mammary glands for the first day or so after birth. It may contain antibodies against diseases previously met or challenged by the dam.

Condition   General health of coat and appearance of the dog.

Conformation   The general make-up of the dog structurally.

Congenital   Deformities/diseases which are present at birth.

Cow hocked   When animal bends his hocks inwards. This is a serious fault.

Cystitis   Inflammation of the bladder.

Dehydration   Loss of water from the tissues which occurs during severe exercise and in various illnesses especially those which produce vomiting and diarrhoea.

Demodectic mange   A parasite which lives deep down in hair follicles.

Dermatitis   Inflammation of the skin – a very complex subject.

Dew claws   Extra claws or functionless digits on the inside of fore and/or hind legs. Usually removed at 3 days.

Diabetes insipidus   A deficiency of the hormone produced by the posterior pituitary gland. It occurs in older dogs and is characterised by the animal's excessive drinking of amounts of water and voiding frequently.

Diabetes mellitus Referred to as 'sweet' or sugar diabetes, this is a disorder of the metabolism of carbohydrates caused by a relative or absolute lack of insulin.

Distemper (hardpad)   An infectious disease in young or older dogs characterised by thick yellow eye and nasal discharges, coughing and thickened pads.

Dominant   Establishing power in genetics.

Dysuria   Difficulty in passing urine (Oliguria = little or no urine).

Eclampsia   A metabolic condition occurring during latter stages of pregnancy or after birth due to a fall in blood sugar/blood calcium levels.

Eczema   A general term for non-contagious skin inflammation characterised by irritation, reddening, sometimes serum and pus. (Wet eczema).

Elizabethan collar   A collar to prevent animal interfering with wounds and dressings.

Encephalitis   Inflammation of specific brain tissue.

Entry form   To be completed when entering a show.

Epizootic   Is a term which applies to a disease which affects a large number of animals in the land and spreads very rapidly.

Extremities   Limbs, ears – peripheral circulation.

Folliculitis   Inflamed hair follicles, which may include demodectic mange.

Gait Movement of the dog.

Gastric dilation/gastric torsion   Abnormal swelling of abdomen due to fermented gas or overeating. Consumption of large amounts of dry food and then large quantities of water make the dog 'swell'. Dogs that gulp food are most susceptible. Immediate action by a vet is absolutely essential.

Haematoma   Injury-related blood-filled space. Aural haematoma is a swelling of the ear causing a blood blister in the ear. (Waxy ears present?)

Haematuria   Any condition in which blood is found in the urine.

Hip dysplasia (H.D.)   Abnormal development of the acetabulum and head of femur (hip joint) leading to abnormal stresses on the ball and socket joint and subsequent possibility of arthritis.

Hormonal imbalance   Poorly controlled abnormal function of certain glands in the endocrine system.

Hydrocephalus   A condition known as water head since a large collection of fluid collects in the brain usually before birth.

Hypertension   High arterial blood pressure.

Idiosyncratic   A reactive peculiarity of an individual dog to a substance absorbed or injected.

Incontinence   Unable to control urine flow.

In-whelp   Pregnant bitch.

Intravenous   An injection used direct into vein.

Isabella   Fawn colour.

Kennel cough   A viral and/or bacterial infection of the upper respiratory tract which is usually very contagious.

Leptospirosis   A bacterial infection that may cause jaundice in dogs. The two types of bacteria affect mainly the liver or kidneys. Recovered dogs may act as carriers of the disease. (*See* Zoonosis)

Level bite   When teeth of the upper and lower incisors meet edge to edge.

Mange   Skin disease caused by parasites. Loss of hair around eyes and face and tips of ears may be a sign of mange. Necessitates early examination by vet for prompt successful treatment. (Skin scrape may be taken).

Mastitis   Inflammation of the mammary glands.

Metabolic   Bio-chemical processes by which the living body is maintained in a stable state by formation and use of essential biochemical substances including energy-rich compounds.

Milk teeth   Puppy teeth.

Mycotic infection   Invasion of living or dead tissue by fungi-Aspergillosis (rhinitis). Rineworm (microsporan, trichophyton outer skin tissue).

Nephritis   Various degrees of renal failure usually associated with noticeable signs of disease (e.g. inappetence, excess thirst, vomiting weight loss, anaemia).

Nephrosis   Gradual debilitating disease of the kidneys associated with generalised oedema of the body.

Non-active register   Animals on this register at the Kennel Club cannot be used for breeding.

Obesity   Overweight. May arise from overfeeding but is often associated with heart disease, arthritis and some skin and respiratory disorders.

Oedema   Fluid accumulation beneath the skin.

Oestrus   Season/heat – 'true' oestrus is where bitch will stand and tie the dog. 'Oestrus cycle' has active and inactive stages and repeats every 6 to 8 months (range 5 to 12 months).

Otitis   Inflammation of the ear. (Otitis Externa – Inflamation of external ear; Otitis Media – Inflammation of middle ear; Otitis Interna – Inflammation of inner ear.)

Overshot   When the front teeth project over and beyond the bottom teeth.

Pancreatic disease   Includes diabetes, infection and tumour formation.

Paraquat   Poison, fatal, with no antidote. Painful, unpleasant and too-frequent cause of death despite veterinary care. Homeopathic treatment would be worth serious consideration if time allows.

Parvo virus   An extremely resistant and pathogenic contagious virus to susceptible animals, especially puppies of under 6 weeks of age.

Pathogen   An organism capable of causing disease.

Pathogenicity   The scale of seriousness of disease caused in a susceptible animal.

Pedigree   A record of the ancestry or line of descent.

Phantom pregnancy   A bitch showing all the signs of a real pregnancy are present in this heartbreaking condition but no puppies are born. Can occur in a bitch who has not been mated.

Placenta   The organ in the mammal by which the foetus is attached to the wall of the uterus and through which it is nourished and waste products are removed frrm it. It leaves the uterus as the 'after birth.'

Psychology   Science of nature and phenomena of the mind.

Puppy   A dog not exceeding twelve months.

Puppy farms   Establishments where whole litters of all breeds of dogs are bought in and sold.

Puppy meal   Small biscuit especially for puppies.

Quality   Superiority of specimen.

Rabies   The most frightening of all dog diseases transmissible to man.

Rickets   The failure of potential new bone in young animals to mineralize due to lack of dietary calcium, limb bones bow and the joints get larger.

Ringworm   A contagious skin disease caused by the growth of certain fungi.

Roundworm   Variably long worms (circular on cross-section) found in the intestine of animals. This word refers to the Ascarid worms of dogs and other domestic pets.

Schedule   Depicts classes held at a dog show.

Scissor bite   When the incisors of the upper jaw just overlap the ones on the bottom jaw.

Season   A term for bitch on heat.

Seborrhoea   An internal disorder of the body as a condition of the skin in which the sebaceous or oil forming glands produce a greasy, dark-smelling coat.

Snipy   A weak narrow muzzle.

Socialisation   Getting puppies used to all environments and situations.

Strychnine   A serious, often fatal poison found in rat poison baits, but one for which treatment can be successful.

Swinging technique   A method of artificial respiration.

Tapeworm   Small or large, flattened, ribbon-like worms which need 2 to 3 hosts and which are of extreme public health importance in certain types.

Temperament   Nature of the dog.

Toxaemia   A presence of toxins (poisons) in the blood stream. Produced by bacteria in the body.

Transgression   To overstep/infringe.

Tuck up   The appearance produced by the abdomen's underline as it sweeps upwards into the flank and/or hindquarter region.

Undershot   Having the lower incisors projected beyond the upper incisors.

Vaccinations   Method of producing active immunity against a specific infection by means of innoculation.

Whelp   A very young puppy.

Whelping   The act of a bitch giving birth.

Whelping Box   Box prepared for bitch to have her puppies in and where the new puppies are kept for the first four weeks of their lives.

Zoonosis   Disease communicable between man and animal (including dog).

Appendix 4

Books for further reading

All about Dog Shows and Showing   D. Cavill
The Book of the Doberman Pinscher   Joan McDonald Brearley
The Complete Doberman Pinscher   Noted Breed Authorities
The Dobermann   Curnow & Faulks
The Dobermann   Hilary Harmer
The Dobermann   Andre Wilhelm
Dog Shows & Show Dogs (A Definitive Study)   Catherine Sutton
Training Dogs   Col. Konrad Most

Index